Innovations in the Management of Foregut Disease

Editor

BRIAN E. LOUIE

THORACIC SURGERY CLINICS

www.thoracic.theclinics.com

Consulting Editor
M. BLAIR MARSHALL

November 2018 • Volume 28 • Number 4

ELSEVIER

1600 John F. Kennedy Boulevard • Suite 1800 • Philadelphia, Pennsylvania, 19103-2899

http://www.thoracic.theclinics.com

THORACIC SURGERY CLINICS Volume 28, Number 4
November 2018 ISSN 1547-4127, ISBN-13: 978-0-323-64134-0

Editor: John Vassallo (j.vassallo@elsevier.com)
Developmental Editor: Laura Fisher

Thoracic Surgery Clinics (ISSN 1547-4127) is published quarterly by Elsevier Inc., 360 Park Avenue South, New York, NY 10010-1710. Months of publication are February, May, August, and November. Business and editorial offices: 1600 John F. Kennedy Boulevard, Suite 1800, Philadelphia, PA 19103-2899. Periodicals postage paid at New York, NY, and additional mailing offices. Subscription prices are $373.00 per year (US individuals), $558.00 per year (US institutions), $100.00 per year (US students), $455.00 per year (Canadian individuals), $721.00 per year (Canadian institutions), $225.00 per year (Canadian and international students), $470.00 per year (international individuals), and $721.00 per year (international institutions). Foreign air speed delivery is included in all Clinics' subscription prices. All prices are subject to change without notice. **POSTMASTER:** Send address changes to Thoracic Surgery Clinics, Elsevier Health Sciences Division, Subscription Customer Service, 3251 Riverport Lane, Maryland Heights, MO 63043. **Customer Service (orders, claims, online, change of address): Telephone: 1-800-654-2452 (U.S. and Canada); 314-447-8871 (outside U.S. and Canada). Fax: 314-447-8029. E-mail: journalscustomerservice-usa@elsevier.com (for print support); journalsonlinesupport-usa@elsevier.com (for online support).**

Reprints. For copies of 100 or more, of articles in this publication, please contact Commercial Rights Department, Elsevier Inc., 360 Park Avenue South, New York, NY 10010-1710. Tel: 212-633-3874; Fax: 212-633-3820; E-mail: reprints@elsevier.com.

Thoracic Surgery Clinics is covered in *MEDLINE/PubMed (Index Medicus), EMBASE/Excerpta Medica, Science Citation Index Expanded (SciSearch®), Journal Citation Reports/Science Edition,* and *Current Contents®/Clinical Medicine.*

Contributors

CONSULTING EDITOR

M. BLAIR MARSHALL, MD, FACS
Chief, Division of Thoracic Surgery, Associate
Professor, Department of Surgery,
Georgetown University Medical Center,
Georgetown University School of Medicine,
Washington, DC, USA

EDITOR

**BRIAN E. LOUIE, MD, MHA, MPH, FRCSC,
FACS**
Director, Thoracic Research and Education,
Executive Co-Medical Director and Surgical
Chair, Swedish Digestive Health Institute,
Co-Director, Minimally Invasive Thoracic
Surgery Program, Division of Thoracic Surgery,
Swedish Cancer Institute, Seattle, Washington,
USA

AUTHORS

RALPH W. AYE, MD, FACS
Program Leader, Thoracic Oncology, Program
Director, Advanced GI, Thoracic Fellowships,
Division of Thoracic Surgery, Swedish Cancer
Institute, Seattle, Washington, USA

SHANDA H. BLACKMON, MD, MPH, FACS
Professor of Surgery, Division of Thoracic
Surgery, Mayo Clinic, Rochester, Minnesota,
USA

STEVEN R. DeMEESTER, MD
Division of Gastrointestinal and Minimally
Invasive Surgery, The Oregon Clinic, The
Foundation for Surgical Innovation and
Education, Portland, Oregon, USA

CHRISTY M. DUNST, MD
Foregut Surgeon, The Oregon Clinic, Portland,
Oregon, USA

ALEXANDER S. FARIVAR, MD
Division of Thoracic Surgery, Swedish Cancer
Institute, Seattle, Washington, USA

ANDREW F. FECZKO, MD
General Surgery Resident, Division of Thoracic
Surgery, Swedish Cancer Institute, Seattle,
Washington, USA

**HIRAN CHRISHANTHA FERNANDO, MBBS,
FRCS, FRCSEd**
Co-Director, Thoracic Oncology, Department
of Surgery, Inova Fairfax Medical Campus,
Falls Church, Virginia, USA

WAYNE L. HOFSTETTER, MD
Professor, Department of Thoracic and
Cardiovascular Surgery, The University of
Texas MD Anderson Cancer Center, Houston,
Texas, USA

ANEE SOPHIA JACKSON, MD
Clinical Research Fellow, Division of Thoracic
Surgery, Swedish Cancer Institute, Seattle,
Washington, USA

BLAIR A. JOBE, MD, FACS
Esophageal and Lung Institute, Allegheny
Health Network, West Penn Hospital,
Pittsburgh, Pennsylvania, USA

YOSHIHIRO KOMATSU, MD
Esophageal and Lung Institute, Allegheny
Health Network, West Penn Hospital,
Pittsburgh, Pennsylvania, USA

JOHN C. LIPHAM, MD
Professor and Chief, Divisions of General and
Minimally Invasive Surgery, Keck School of
Medicine of USC, University of Southern
California, Los Angeles, California,
USA

**BRIAN E. LOUIE, MD, MHA, MPH, FRCSC,
FACS**
Director, Thoracic Research and Education,
Executive Co-Medical Director and Surgical
Chair, Swedish Digestive Health Institute,
Co-Director, Minimally Invasive Thoracic
Surgery Program, Division of Thoracic Surgery,
Swedish Cancer Institute, Seattle, Washington,
USA

JAMES D. LUKETICH, MD
Henry T. Bahnson Professor of Cardiothoracic
Surgery, Chair, Department of Cardiothoracic
Surgery, Chief, Division of Thoracic and
Foregut Surgery, Director, Thoracic Surgical
Oncology, Director, UPMC Esophageal and
Lung Surgery Institute, Director, Mark
Ravitch/Leon C. Hirsch Center for Minimally
Invasive Surgery, University of Pittsburgh
Medical Center, Pittsburgh, Pennsylvania,
USA

MARISSA ANNE MAYOR, MD
Surgical Resident, Department of Surgery,
Inova Fairfax Medical Campus, Falls Church,
Virginia, USA

DANIELA R. MOLENA, MD, FACS
Associate Professor, Thoracic Surgery Service,
Memorial Sloan Kettering Cancer Center,
New York, New York, USA

KIRSTEN M. NEWHAMS, MD, MPH
Esophageal and Lung Institute, Allegheny
Health Network, West Penn Hospital,
Pittsburgh, Pennsylvania, USA

RAVI RAJARAM, MD, MSc
Cardiothoracic Surgery Fellow, Department of
Thoracic and Cardiovascular Surgery, The
University of Texas MD Anderson Cancer
Center, Houston, Texas, USA

MATTHEW ROCHEFORT, MD
Division of Thoracic Surgery, Brigham and
Women's Hospital, Boston, Massachusetts,
USA

MANUEL VILLA SANCHEZ, MD
Assistant Professor, Department of
Cardiothoracic Surgery, University of
Pittsburgh Medical Center, Pittsburgh,
Pennsylvania, USA

LARA W. SCHAHEEN, MD
Resident, Department of Cardiothoracic
Surgery, University of Pittsburgh Medical
Center, Pittsburgh, Pennsylvania,
USA

MONISHA SUDARSHAN, MD, MPH
Division of Thoracic Surgery, Mayo Clinic,
Rochester, Minnesota, USA

JAMES M. TATUM, MD
Clinical Instructor, Department of Surgery,
Division of General and Laparoscopic Surgery,
Keck School of Medicine of USC, University of
Southern California, Los Angeles, California,
USA

EZRA N. TEITELBAUM, MD, MEd
Assistant Professor of Surgery and Medical
Education, Northwestern University Feinberg
School of Medicine, Chicago, Illinois,
USA

SIMON R. TURNER, MD, MEd, FRCSC
Assistant Professor, Division of Thoracic
Surgery, University of Alberta, Edmonton,
Alberta, Canada

JEFFREY R. WATKINS, MD
Division of Thoracic Surgery, Swedish Cancer
Institute, Seattle, Washington, USA

JON O. WEE, MD
Section Chief, Esophageal Surgery,
Co-Director of Minimally Invasive Thoracic
Surgery, Director of Robotics in Thoracic
Surgery, Division of Thoracic Surgery, Brigham
and Women's Hospital, Boston,
Massachusetts, USA

AHMED M. ZIHNI, MD, MPH
Division of Gastrointestinal and Minimally
Invasive Surgery, The Oregon Clinic,
Providence Portland Medical Center,
The Foundation for Surgical Innovation
and Education, Portland, Oregon,
USA

Contents

> Peroral endoscopic myotomy surgery is an incisionless, minimally invasive, natural orifice technique used to treat the symptoms of achalasia and other spastic disorders of the esophagus. Recent experience demonstrates that it can be performed safely by experienced esophageal surgeons, and there are very good short-term outcomes comparable with laparoscopic myotomy. The rapid worldwide adoption of this technique demonstrates its potential to replace the current therapies available for achalasia. A cautionary note is important in that long-term outcomes are not yet available in terms of dysphagia and gastroesophageal reflux disease symptoms.

> Endoscopic cricopharyngeal myotomy has been demonstrated to be a safe and efficacious procedure with favorable outcomes for the treatment of cricopharyngeal dysfunction with or without Zenker diverticulum. It is a less invasive approach with decreased morbidity compared with the open approach and minimal reported complications. Peroral endoscopic pyloromyotomy is a novel technique for the treatment of gastroparesis. It has shown promising results in terms of its safety, complication profile, and symptom improvement in a minimally invasive approach that is appealing to many patients. As further data emerge on the technique, long-term efficacy of the procedure will be better understood.

> Gastroesophageal reflux disease (GERD) is a common affliction in Western society. In patients in whom GERD is resistant to medical therapy or who desire nonpharmacologic definitive therapy, several surgical interventions are available. The most common and traditional surgical therapy is partial or complete gastric fundoplication; however, new alternatives, including the magnetic augmentation system LINX and EndoStim device, are increasingly common and efficacious.

> Endoluminal antireflux procedures were pioneered in the 1980s as an alternative to the more invasive Nissen fundoplication. Recent advances in device design and technique have generated renewed interest. Herein the authors review available data for currently available devices used for endoluminal therapy for gastroesophageal reflux disease.

> The ideal operative solution to giant paraesophageal hernias involves a complex evaluation of the functional anatomy and the intraoperative assessment of both esophageal length and crural closure tension. The addition of surgical adjuncts such as extended transmediastinal dissection, Collis gastroplasty, and mesh reinforcement are all necessary, on an individualized basis, to address these 2 primary causes of hernia recurrence. The authors discuss the options available.

Esophageal perforation has historically been a devastating condition resulting in high morbidity and mortality. The use of endoluminal therapies to treat esophageal leaks and perforations has grown exponentially over the last decade and offers many advantages over traditional surgical intervention in the appropriate circumstances. New interventional endoscopic techniques, including endoscopic clips, covered metal stents, and endoluminal vacuum therapy, have been developed over the last several years to manage esophageal perforation in an attempt to decrease the related morbidity and mortality.

The understanding of esophageal function and dysfunction in a variety of disease states has largely been driven by the introduction of measurement technologies. Included in these are contrast esophagram, computed tomography, high-resolution manometry, and 24-hour pH monitoring. Two novel measurement technologies, the functional lumen imaging probe and mucosal impedance catheter, have recently been introduced and studied. This article discusses the technological basis of these tools and the evidence behind their application in the measurement of esophageal anatomy, physiology, and histology pertaining to several diseases, including gastroesophageal reflux disease, achalasia, and eosinophilic esophagitis.

Intraoperative fluorescence imaging (FI) with indocyanine green has several potential uses during esophagectomy. Intravascular injection for enhancing the visualization of conduit vascularity and assessing macroperfusion and microperfusion has the most literature support and may help reduce anastomotic leaks. Peritumoral injection has been reported for use in identifying sentinel nodes during lymphadenectomy, and intralymphatic injection may be used to help preserve or ligate the thoracic duct. The authors' own technique of FI for conduit assessment is described. They routinely use this strategy to guide anastomosis placement and reduce leaks.

Adoption of new practices is challenging to the surgeon innovator given the lack of standardized processes for implementation. Credentialed surgeons who want to apply new practices need to ensure adequate training depending on the procedure and underlying skills. A competent and motivated team needs to be identified and appropriate privileging sought for the procedure from the local institution. Planning for meticulous monitoring of outcomes ensures continuous safety and quality surveillance. Patients need complete transparency when being informed about a novel practice with information on comparison with standard-of-care treatments.

THORACIC SURGERY CLINICS

SERIES OF RELATED INTEREST

Surgical Clinics
available at: http://www.surgical.theclinics.com
Surgical Oncology Clinics
available at: http://www.surgonc.theclinics.com
Advances in Surgery
available at: http://www.advancessurgery.com

THE CLINICS ARE AVAILABLE ONLINE!
Access your subscription at:
www.theclinics.com

Erratum

The Karolinska Institutet found that the research reported in the paper "Airway transplantation," co-authored by Philipp Jungebluth and Paolo Macchiarini, and published in the February 2014 issue of *Thoracic Surgery Clinics* (Volume 24, issue 1, pages 97-106) constitutes scientific misconduct. This article has been retracted at the request of the Karolinska Institutet. In this paper, data from clinical research are reported in Table 3. The Karolinska Institutet concluded that no ethical permit had been obtained for the underlying clinical research regarding the patients reported from Karolinska. The research was carried out without sufficient support by preclinical data. The paper presents its data in a way that is unduly positive and uncritical. The clinical findings reported are not supported by source data.

Thorac Surg Clin 28 (2018) xi
https://doi.org/10.1016/j.thorsurg.2018.08.001

Preface

Innovations in and Around the Foregut

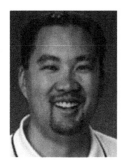

Brian E. Louie, MD, MHA, MPH, FRCSC, FACS
Editor

The esophagus has a deceptively simple role in the human body: deliver orally ingested material from the mouth to the stomach. Yet, it is involved in and the source of much disease from the highly prevalent gastroesophageal reflux (GERD) to the more rare motility disorders such as achalasia, and last, the Barrett-adenocarcinoma pathway. Over the last several years, considerable progress and changes in diagnostic tools and approaches to surgical treatments of esophageal disease have been made. In this issue of *Thoracic Surgery Clinics*, we examine a cadre of new innovations and some that have been around for some time.

The first content theme surrounds the management of Barrett esophagus. Diagnosis has evolved from endoscopic biopsies using the Seattle protocol with new diagnostic tools, such as wide area transepithelial sampling, optical coherence tomography, and confocal laser endomicroscopy to enhance the detection and diagnosis of Barrett esophagus along the continuum from nondysplastic to dysplasia. With early detection, subsequent treatment before cancer has developed can be initiated and involve endoscopic resections and ablative therapies.

Open operations gave way to laparoscopic approaches, and we are witnessing another paradigm shift as endoscopic surgery takes us into the potential space of the submucosa: the highway of the esophagus. Per oral endoscopic myotomy has been rapidly adopted around the world as an alternative to laparoscopic myotomy. This has also opened up additional options to address diseases related to the cricopharyngeal muscle (Zenker diverticulum) and the pylorus (gastroparesis) with flexible endoscopy.

Nissen fundoplication and its modifications have been the only surgical option for the management of GERD for 70 years. The surgical armamentarium for GERD has more than doubled with viable options that focus on restoring the LES function and seek to balance the control of GERD with the potential side effects of Nissen. The procedures involve extraluminal devices, such as magnetic sphincter augmentation and electrical stimulation of the lower esophageal sphincter, and endoluminal approaches, like transoral incisionless fundoplication. The difficult hiatus during repair of the large hiatal hernia remains a challenge as evidenced by high recurrence rates. Surgical adjuncts, such as mesh, gastroplasty, and relaxing incisions, have been added to simple suture closure to mitigate against the tensions found at the esophageal hiatus during repair.

Even the management of perforations and anastomotic problems has moved endoluminal. Most thoracic surgeons are acquainted with the use of clips and stents, but the use of endoluminal wound vacuum therapy has emerged as a viable option to not only stents, but also diversion and exclusion.

Poised to influence the diagnosis and treatment of esophageal diseases are the functional endoluminal probes that may guide therapy in achalasia or esophageal tissue impedance as a new diagnostic test for GERD.

The problem of gastric pull-up perfusion during esophagectomy is delineated by the use of fluorescence imaging and can be used to select an

Thorac Surg Clin 28 (2018) xiii–xiv
https://doi.org/10.1016/j.thorsurg.2018.08.002
1547-4127/18/© 2018 Published by Elsevier Inc.

thoracic.theclinics.com

appropriately vascularized location for the esophagogastric anastomosis in hopes of lowering the anastomotic complication rate.

Last, a careful look at how the adoption and integration of these new techniques into clinical practice in terms of training, credentialing, and evaluation should occur is examined.

I want to thank all the authors for their time and contributions to this issue of *Thoracic Surgery Clinics*. I hope that you'll enjoy reviewing these articles and find something that is innovative that can be useful in your thoracic surgical practice.

Brian E. Louie, MD, MHA, MPH, FRCSC, FACS
Division of Thoracic Surgery
Swedish Cancer Institute
Suite 900
1101 Madison Street
Seattle, WA 98104, USA

E-mail address:
brian.louie@swedish.org

Enhancing the Detection of Barrett Esophagus

Yoshihiro Komatsu, MD, Kirsten M. Newhams, MD, MPH, Blair A. Jobe, MD*

KEYWORDS

- Barrett esophagus • Neoplasia • Endoscopic imaging • Narrow band imaging
- Wide area transepithelial sampling with 3-dimensional analysis • Transnasal endoscopy

KEY POINTS

- The incidence of esophageal adenocarcinoma and its premalignant condition, Barrett esophagus (BE), has increased.
- Screening for BE is not recommended in general population. Surveillance endoscopy is recommended in patients with BE.
- Endoscopy with the Seattle protocol is the standard approach for BE surveillance.
- Advanced imaging techniques may enable targeted biopsies to improve the accuracy of BE surveillance.

INTRODUCTION

Barrett esophagus (BE) is defined as the replacement of normal squamous epithelium with metaplastic columnar epithelium with goblet cells.[1,2] This inflammatory condition is a result of chronic exposure of the esophageal epithelium to refluxed gastric contents. Gastroesophageal reflux disease (GERD) is an increasingly prevalent disease, especially in Western countries. BE is a known major risk factor for the development of esophageal adenocarcinoma (EAC), the incidence of which has increased dramatically since the 1970s.[3–5] The risk of developing EAC among patients with BE is 30- to 125-fold higher compared with the general population.[6] Ultimately, few patients with BE develop EAC, with an annual risk of 0.1% to 0.5%.[7,8] Individuals with BE are often asymptomatic and therefore are not selected for screening, leading to uncertain prevalence and incidence. Based on current studies, the prevalence of BE has been estimated to be about 2% among patients who have undergone upper endoscopy for any reason. The incidence of BE among patients with GERD symptoms varies between 5% and 20%.[1,9–11] The increased incidence of BE is thought to be caused by increasing availability and frequency of endoscopy.[12]

The endoscopist has a critical role of suspecting the presence of BE and obtaining tissue to confirm a diagnosis. A key component of this skill is considering risk factors such as GERD, obesity, family history, and tobacco use.

Generally, BE is suspected when columnar epithelium (ie, pink salmon-colored epithelium) is observed endoscopically to extend proximal to the gastroesophageal junction (GEJ) into the esophagus. Currently, there are 2 different landmarks to identify the GEJ. The most proximal extent of the gastric folds is used as the landmark in Western countries, while the most distal extent of palisade vessels is used as the landmark in Asian countries. Most published data on BE use the proximal extent of gastric folds as the

Disclosure: The authors have nothing to disclose.
Esophageal and Lung Institute, Allegheny Health Network, Western Pennsylvania Hospital, Suite 158, Mellon Pavilion, 4815 Liberty Avenue, Pittsburgh, PA 15224, USA
* Corresponding author.
E-mail address: Blair.JOBE@ahn.org

Thorac Surg Clin 28 (2018) 453–464
https://doi.org/10.1016/j.thorsurg.2018.07.011

landmark of GEJ. The location of the most proximal extent of gastric folds may be affected by distension of the esophagus and stomach, respiration, and gastric motility. The GEJ should be measured when the stomach is decompressed so that the gastric folds are most visible.

Once BE has been identified, it can be divided into short segment or long segment based on the extent of changes. BE that is less than 3 cm is considered short segment, while BE that is longer than 3 cm is considered long segment.[13] The risk of cancer in BE increases with the length of esophageal metaplasia.[14] Currently, the Prague circumferential (C) and maximal extent (M) classification often is used to objectively describe the extent of BE.[15] This classification is valuable in objectively describing a patient's BE as well as directing treatment and follow-up.

The definitive diagnosis of BE is made pathologically by the presence of intestinal metaplasia on an esophageal biopsy. Endoscopic surveillance has been proposed for patients with BE in order to detect dysplasia and neoplasia in an early stage. Although it remains uncertain if endoscopic surveillance of patients with BE reduces mortality from esophageal adenocarcinoma, current guidelines recommend endoscopic surveillance at 3 to 5 year intervals for BE without dysplasia, 6 to 12 months for those with low-grade dysplasia, and every 3 months for those with high-grade dysplasia who do not undergo intervention.[16]

SEATTLE PROTOCOL

The goal of surveillance of patients with BE is to prevent the evolution or progression of adenocarcinoma. The Seattle protocol is used to detect dysplasia and neoplasia by obtaining 4-quadrant biopsy sampling at 1 to 2 cm intervals throughout the area of suspected BE. The intention of the Seattle protocol is to increase the chance of identifying dysplasia and neoplasia that may be randomly distributed throughout the area of BE. In addition to Seattle protocol sampling, targeted biopsies should be performed of mucosal irregularities, such as nodules, masses, and ulcerations. The sensitivity of this protocol is diminished because of sampling error, especially for long segment disease where dysplastic and neoplastic lesions tend to have patchy and focal distribution[17–20] (**Fig. 1**). Early studies demonstrated foci of unsuspected carcinoma in up to 73% of resected esophagectomy specimens for high-grade dysplasia.[19] It has been reported that random biopsies obtained with white light endoscopy sample only 4% to 5% of Barrett

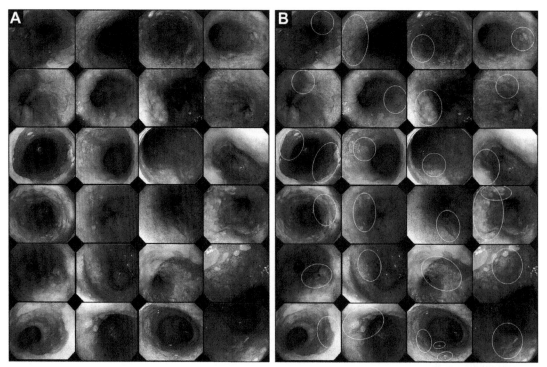

Fig. 1. (*A*) Examples of subtle neoplastic lesions in BE. (*B*) The neoplastic lesions are indicated with circles. (*From* Boerwinkel DF, Swager AF, Curvers WL, et al. The clinical consequences of advanced imaging techniques in Barrett esophagus. Gastroenterology 2014;146(3):623; with permission.)

epithelium.[21,22] In order to improve the accuracy of endoscopic surveillance for BE, advanced imaging and targeted biopsy techniques should be considered.

CHROMOENDOSCOPY

Chromoendoscopy is an advanced technique to improve mucosal visualization. It consists of spraying the mucosa with a chemical solution to enhance visualization of the mucosal surface as well as the vascular pattern of absorption. Chemical solutions that have been described include indigo carmine, methylene blue, and acetic acid.[23,24]

Compared with other novel imaging technology, chromoendoscopy is relatively inexpensive and readily available. The disadvantages of chromoendoscopy include its use of a staining agent and spraying catheter; its labor-intensive nature, sometimes requiring multiple sprays and lavage for optimal imaging; and high interobserver variability in the ability to identify abnormal areas.[23]

Indigo carmine is a nonabsorptive contrast dye that pools in the mucosal grooves and pits that enhances the mucosal irregularities and topographic visualization. Sharma and colleagues[25] proposed 3 different mucosal patterns in BE after indigo carmine chromoendoscopy and inspection with magnification endoscopy: circular, ridged/villous, and irregular/distorted pattern. Ridged/villous pattern is associated with intestinal metaplasia, and irregular/distorted pattern is associated with dysplasia and neoplasia.

Methylene blue is absorbed by certain tissues including intestinal epithelium, but it is not absorbed by squamous or gastric epithelium. Abnormal absorptive mucosa in BE will be stained blue, and the normal mucosa will not be stained (**Fig. 2**). The pattern of stain for dysplasia and neoplasia differs within BE.[26] Dysplastic/neoplastic mucosa is more weakly stained or unstained, allowing targeted biopsies.[27] A recent meta-analysis of 9 studies demonstrated that there is no incremental yield for methylene blue chromoendoscopy over white light endoscopy.[28]

Another option for advanced imaging techniques uses acetic acid. Acetic acid provides increased contrast enhancement of the mucosa when used in combination with magnification endoscopy and high-resolution white light endoscopy.[29–31] After applying acetic acid, normal squamous epithelium becomes white, while Barrett esophageal mucosa and gastric columnar mucosa become white initially but turn red after 2 to 3 minutes[32] (**Figs. 3** and **4**). A meta-analysis of 8 prospective studies demonstrated that the pooled sensitivity and specificity for detecting BE with acetic acid enhancement were 96% and 69%, respectively.[33] Acetic acid chromoendoscopy for BE has a stated benefit of increased detection of dysplasia and neoplasia. In the same study, the pooled sensitivity and specificity for the diagnosis of high grade dysplasia and neoplasia were 92% and 96%, respectively.[33] In a retrospective study of 982 patients with BE undergoing surveillance, Tholoor and colleagues[34] demonstrated that targeted biopsy with acetic acid chromoendoscopy showed a higher rate of detection of dysplasia

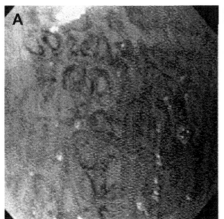
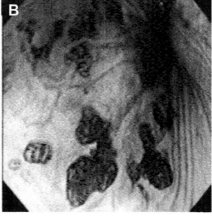

Fig. 2. Endoscopic high-magnification image of Barrett mucosa after methylene blue staining showing a tubular mucosal pit pattern. (*A*) Magnification to approximately 115 × (Olympus 160Z high-magnification endoscope; Olympus America), (*B*) Magnification to approximately 115 × (Olympus 240Z high-magnification endoscope; Olympus America). (*From* Canto MI. Chromoendoscopy and magnifying endoscopy for Barrett's esophagus. Clin Gastroenterol Hepatol 2005;3(7 Suppl 1):S13; with permission.)

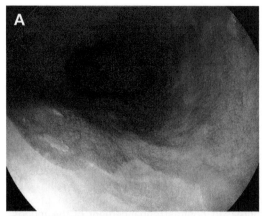

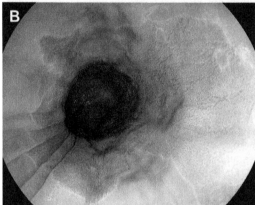

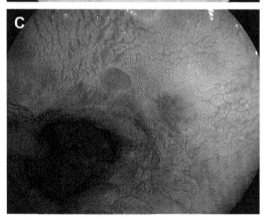

Fig. 3. (*A*) NDBE on WLE. (*B*) NDBE on acetic acid chromoendoscopy. (*C*) Focal loss of acetowhitening (erythematous patch) indicating a dysplastic focus in BE. BE, Barrett esophagus; NDBE, nondysplastic Barrett esophagus; WLE, white-light endoscopy. (*From* Tholoor S, Bhattacharyya R, Tsagkournis O, et al. Acetic acid chromoendoscopy in Barrett's esophagus surveillance is superior to the standardized random biopsy protocol: results from a large cohort study (with video). Gastrointest Endosc 2014;80(3):419; with permission.)

and neoplasia when compared with the random biopsy group (13% and 2%, respectively). Furthermore, using acetic acid has a lower number of biopsies needed to detect 1 patient with dysplasia and neoplasia when compared with a random biopsy group (40 and 604, respectively).[34] Recent studies have suggested that acetic acid chromoendoscopy may be beneficial for identification of early neoplasia.[35,36] Further confirmation with randomized crossover trials should be considered.

ELECTRONIC CHROMOENDOSCOPY

Electronic chromoendoscopy refers to novel endoscopic imaging technologies that provide detailed contrast enhancement of the mucosal surface and blood vessels including narrow band imaging (NBI) (Olympus Medical Systems, Tokyo, Japan), flexible spectral imaging color enhancement (FICE) (Fujinon, Fujifilm Medical Company, Saitama, Japan), and i-SCAN (PENTAX Endoscopy, Tokyo, Japan). As interaction of particular tissue structures with light depends on wavelength, enhancement of certain mucosal structures with electronic chromoendoscopy may be achieved by light transmission at selected wavelengths.[37] Selective light transmittance is achieved by optical filtering of white light in NBI, whereas FICE and i-SCAN accomplish this via software after imaging processing[20] (**Fig. 5**).

Narrow Band Imaging

NBI is based on the phenomenon that depth of light penetration depends on the light wavelength.[38] A shorter wavelength (blue light) penetrates superficially into the mucosa, whereas a longer wavelength (red light) penetrates deeper into tissue. The light from a xenon arc lamp through the NBI filter produces 2 narrow bands of light centered at the specific wavelengths of 415 nm and 540 nm. These 2 wavelengths correspond to the primary and secondary light absorption peaks of hemoglobin, respectively.[39] The effect of NBI on mucosa emphasizes the blood vessels in sharp contrast within the nonvascular structures, because most of the NBI light is absorbed by the blood vessels, resulting in better visualization of vascular structures.

Flexible Spectral Imaging Color Enhancement and i-SCAN

FICE is a proprietary digital imaging postprocessing system of Fujinon and uses a white light endoscopic image that is mathematically processed by emphasizing certain ranges of wavelengths. Three single wavelengths, including red, green, and blue, can be selected to demonstrate a composite

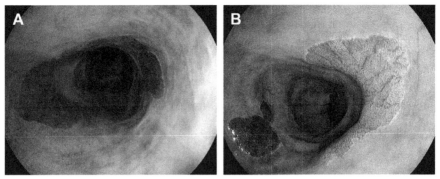

Fig. 4. (*A*) NDBE on WLE (*B*) Same patient as 2A after acetic acid chromoendoscopy showing normal Barrett island on the right and dysplastic island (loss of acetowhitening) on the left. (*From* Tholoor S, Bhattacharyya R, Tsagkournis O, et al. Acetic acid chromoendoscopy in Barrett's esophagus surveillance is superior to the standardized random biopsy protocol: results from a large cohort study (with video). Gastrointest Endosc 2014;80(3):420; with permission.)

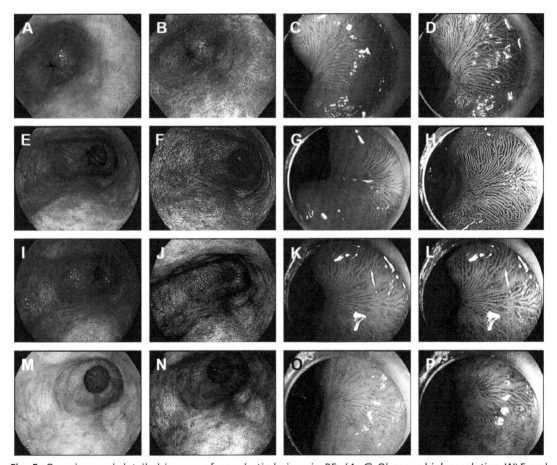

Fig. 5. Overview and detailed images of neoplastic lesions in BE. (*A, C*) Olympus high-resolution WLE and (*B, D*) NBI, (*E, G*) Fujinon WLE and (*F, H*) BLI, (*I, K*) Fujinon WLE and (*J, L*) Fuji Intelligent Chromo Endoscopy, and (*M, O*) Pentax WLE and (*N, P*) i-scan. BE, Barrett esophagus; BLI, blue laser imaging; NBI, narrow band imaging; WLE, white light endoscopy. (*From* Boerwinkel DF, Swager AF, Curvers WL, et al. The clinical consequences of advanced imaging techniques in Barrett's esophagus. Gastroenterology 2014;146(3):624; with permission.)

color-enhanced image in real time. The optimal FICE setting for tissue diagnosis has not been established.

i-SCAN is another software-driven postprocessing image enhancement technology from PENTAX Endoscopy using white light endoscopic image similar to FICE.

Clinical Use of Electronic Chromoendoscopy

NBI has been the most studied electronic chromoendoscopy with BE. NBI enhances visualization of esophageal mucosa and can potentially detect BE and associated dysplasia and neoplasia.[40–42] Regular vascular and mucosal NBI patterns have shown correlation with nondysplastic Barrett's esophageal mucosa, whereas irregular patterns have demonstrated an association with dysplasia and neoplasia.[38,43] Several studies have proposed classification systems using NBI for BE.[25,43–46] None of them have been accepted because of unsatisfactory validation studies and their complex and impractical nature in the clinical setting.[47–50] Recently, the Barrett's International NBI Group (BING) designed a consensus-driven BING-criteria NBI classification system.[51] These criteria are using simpler surface and vascular patterns to predict the presence of metaplasia, dysplasia, and neoplasia. Mucosal and vascular patterns in NBI imaging are classified as regular or irregular based on morphologic characteristics agreed on by BING (**Table 1**). Regular

mucosal patterns are defined by circular, ridged/villous, or tubular patterns being arranged in orderly fashion; irregular mucosal patterns are defined by absent or irregular surface patterns (**Fig. 6**). Regular vascular patterns are marked by blood vessels situated regularly along or between mucosal ridges and/or those showing normal, long, branching patterns, whereas irregular vascular patterns are marked by focally or diffusely distributed vessels not following the normal architecture of mucosa (**Fig. 7**). Regular mucosal and vascular patterns were predictive of nondysplastic BE, whereas irregular patterns were predictive of dysplasia and neoplasia. Compared with previously proposed classification systems, the BING version is simpler and easier to implement in a clinical setting, with high levels of accuracy and interobserver agreement.[51]

WIDE AREA TRANSEPITHELIAL SAMPLING WITH 3-DIMENSIONAL TISSUE ANALYSIS

Wide area transepithelial sampling with 3-dimensional tissue analysis (WATS^{3D}, CDx Diagnostics, New York) is a new endoscopic sampling technique that uses a special abrasive brushing instrument to obtain tissue samples from a broad area of BE (**Fig. 8**). Traditionally, BE has been surveilled using the Seattle protocol, which samples about 4% to 5% of an area of BE.[21,22] WATS^{3D} was created to obtain a larger tissue sample from an area of suspected or established BE. Sampled tissue is computer-analyzed to identify the most suspicious cells for review by the pathologist. A multicenter prospective randomized trial was conducted with 160 patients with BE to compare detection of advanced disease between WATS^{3D} in combination with Seattle protocol and Seattle protocol alone.[52] This study demonstrated that the use of WATS^{3D} in combination of Seattle protocol was able to detect more cases of high-grade dysplasia and neoplasia than the Seattle protocol alone. The Seattle protocol alone detected 7 cases of high-grade dysplasia and neoplasia, while WATS^{3D} revealed 23 more cases of high-grade dysplasia and neoplasia that were not detected by Seattle protocol alone.[52] Another prospective study with a larger cohort of patients with BE was conducted by the US collaborative WATS3D study group.[53] This study enrolled more than 4000 patients with suspected or established BE. The patients either underwent screening endoscopy with Seattle protocol alone or Seattle protocol with WATS^{3D}. BE was detected in 594 patients by Seattle protocol alone and in 799 patients by WATS^{3D}. Of the

Table 1 Consensus-driven narrow band imaging classification of Barrett epithelium	
Morphologic Characteristics	**Classification**
Mucosal pattern	
Circular, ridged/villous, or tubular patterns	Regular
Absent or irregular patterns	Irregular
Vascular pattern	
Blood vessels situated regularly along or between mucosal ridges and/or those showing normal, long, branching patterns	Regular
Focally or diffusely distributed vessels not following normal architecture of the mucosa	Irregular

From Sharma P, Bergman JJ, Goda K, et al. Development and validation of a classification system to identify high-grade dysplasia and esophageal adenocarcinoma in Barrett's esophagus using narrow-band imaging. Gastroenterology 2016;150(3):592; with permission.

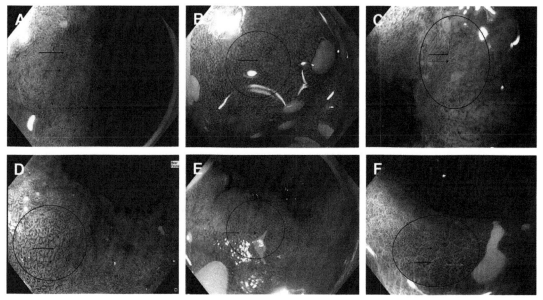

Fig. 6. (*A*) High-resolution images of NDBE using NBI. Note the presence of circular mucosal patterns (*solid arrow*) that are arranged in an orderly fashion and blood vessels that clearly follow the mucosal architecture (*dashed arrow*). (*B*) High-resolution images of NDBE using NBI. Note the presence of circular mucosal patterns that are arranged in an orderly fashion and blood vessels that clearly follow the normal architecture of mucosa (*solid arrow*). (*C*) High-resolution images of NDBE using NBI. Note the presence of circular mucosal patterns (*solid arrow*) that are arranged in an orderly fashion and blood vessels that clearly follow the architecture of the mucosal ridges (*dashed arrow*). (*D*) High-resolution images of NDBE using NBI. Note the presence of ridge/villous mucosal patterns (*solid arrow*) that are arranged in an orderly fashion and blood vessels that are arranged in a regular fashion between the mucosal ridges (*dashed arrows*). (*E*) High-resolution images of NDBE using NBI. Note the presence of circular mucosal patterns (*solid arrow*) that are arranged in an orderly fashion and blood vessels that follow the architecture of the mucosa (*dashed arrow*). (*F*) High-resolution images of NDBE using NBI. Note the presence of circular (*solid black arrow*) and ridge/villous (*red arrow*) mucosal patterns arranged in an orderly fashion and blood vessels that follow the mucosal ridge architecture (*dashed arrow*). (*From* Sharma P, Bergman JJ, Goda K, et al. Development and validation of a classification system to identify high-grade dysplasia and esophageal adenocarcinoma in Barrett's esophagus using narrow-band imaging. Gastroenterology 2016;150(3):593; with permission.)

799 patients with BE detected by WATS[3D], 493 were not diagnosed with BE by Seattle protocol. Therefore, the addition of the WATS[3D] increased the detection of BE by 83% (493/594; 95% confidence interval [CI] 74%–93%). The additional detection of BE in 12% of all patients tested with WATS (494/4203) results in the number of patients needed to screen to detect one additional case of BE of 8.53. In addition, low-grade dysplasia was detected in 26 patients by Seattle protocol alone and in 33 patients by Seattle protocol with WATS[3D]. Of the 33 patients diagnosed with low-grade dysplasia, 23 had negative results for low-grade dysplasia by Seattle protocol alone. The addition of WATS[3D] to Seattle protocol increased the detection of LGD by 88.5% (23/26; 95% CI 48%–160%).[53] These results suggest that the implementation of WATS[3D] may improve surveillance of BE.

CYTOSPONGE™

Cytosponge™ (Medtronic, Minneapolis, Minnesota) is a novel technique of esophageal sampling to screen BE, dysplasia, and carcinoma of the esophagus. Cytosponge™ is a nonendoscopic, ingestible sampling device consisting of a gelatin capsule on a string that dissolves in the stomach (**Fig. 9**). When the capsule dissolves, a small sponge inside of the capsule expands in the stomach and is drawn out of mouth by pulling the string, collecting esophageal cells in the process. The procedure takes 5 minutes to complete. Immunohistochemistry on the sponge is performed to identify the biomarker for BE, trefoil factor 3 (TFF3), which helps in distinguishing BE from the gastric cardia and squamous cells of the esophagus and larynx.[54]

Several studies have shown the acceptability and accuracy of the Cytosponge™ TFF3 test for

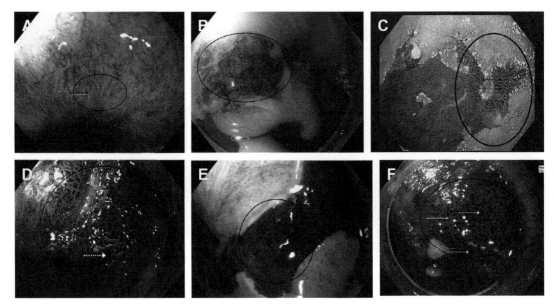

Fig. 7. (*A*) High-resolution images of dysplastic BE using NBI. Irregular mucosal and vascular patterns in BE patient using NBI. Note the irregular mucosal (*black arrow*) and vascular patterns (*red arrow*). (*B*) High-resolution images of dysplastic BE using NBI. Irregular mucosal and vascular patterns in BE patient using NBI. Note the irregular mucosal (*black arrow*) and vascular patterns (*red arrow*). The vessels do not follow the normal architecture of the mucosa. (*C*) High-resolution images of dysplastic BE using NBI. Irregular mucosal and vascular patterns in BE patient using NBI. Note the irregular mucosal (*solid black arrow*) and vascular patterns (*dashed arrow*). In contrast, red arrow shows area on the mucosa where vessels are arranged in a regular fashion that follows the normal architecture of the mucosa. (*D*) High-resolution images of dysplastic BE using NBI. Irregular mucosal and vascular patterns in BE patient using NBI (*black arrow*). Note the irregular mucosal and vascular patterns (*dashed arrow*). The focally or diffusely distributed vessels do not follow the normal architecture of the mucosa. (*E*) High-resolution images of dysplastic BE using NBI. Irregular mucosal and vascular patterns in BE patient using NBI. Note the irregular mucosal and vascular patterns (*solid arrow*); the dashed arrow in contrast show regularly arranged mucosal and vascular pattern. (*F*) High-resolution images of dysplastic BE using NBI. Irregular mucosal and vascular patterns in BE patient using NBI. Note the irregular mucosal (*solid arrow*) and vascular patterns (*dashed arrows*). (*From* Sharma P, Bergman JJ, Goda K, et al. Development and validation of a classification system to identify high-grade dysplasia and esophageal adenocarcinoma in Barrett's esophagus using narrow-band imaging. Gastroenterology 2016;150(3):594; with permission.)

screening for BE.[55,56] The BE Screening Trial 1 (BEST1) is a cohort study involved 501 patients with previous prescriptions for acid suppression medications in the United Kingdom primary care setting that demonstrated Cytosponge™ with TFF3 IHC had sensitivity and specificity of 73% and 94%, respectively for short segment BE (<2 cm circumferential), which further increased to 90% and 93.5%, respectively for longer BE (>2 cm circumferential).[55] Subsequently, in the BE Screening Trial 2 (BEST2) a case-control study was conducted to evaluate 1110 patients who underwent evaluation by both Cytosponge™ and endoscopy.[56] The Cytosponge™ procedure was successfully performed on 94% of patients. The overall sensitivity and specificity of BE diagnosis by Cytosponge™ for short segment BE (<3 cm) were 80% and 92%, respectively. Furthermore, the sensitivity was increased to 87% in patients with long-segment BE (>3 cm) and to 89% in

patients who swallowed Cytosponge™ twice during the study period.[56] Benaglia and colleagues[57] demonstrated that Cytosponge™ screening followed by endoscopic treatment was more cost-effective than endoscopic screening and treatment. Cytosponge™ is not available in the United States yet. Because of its simplicity and cost-effectiveness, the Cytosponge™ has potential to be an alternative screening method for detecting BE.

TRANSNASAL ENDOSCOPY

Transnasal endoscopy is performed in an outpatient clinic setting using an ultrathin endoscope through the nares following the application of a topical anesthetic agent without sedation. With the lack of anesthesia and ease of use, transnasal endoscopy could potentially reduce the cost of BE screening when compared with a sedated

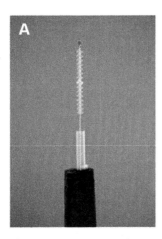

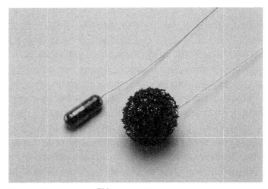

Fig. 9. Cytosponge™ in gelatin capsule and expanded cytosponge. (*Courtesy of* Medtronic, Minneapolis, MN; with permission.)

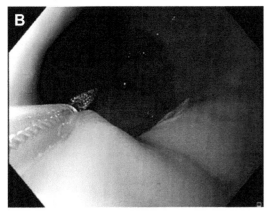

Fig. 8. (*A*) WATS[3D] abrasive brushing instrument. (*B*) Endoscopic view of brushing instrument and esophagus. Unlike traditional cytology instruments, which obtain only superficial exfoliated cells, WATS[3D] uses an abrasive brush that samples the full-thickness epithelium and was designed to consistently sample deeper layers of the more firmly attached glandular epithelium found in Barrett esophagus. (*From* Gross SA, Smith MS, Kaul V, et al. Increased detection of Barrett's esophagus and esophageal dysplasia with adjunctive use of wide-area transepithelial sample with three-dimensional computer-assisted analysis (WATS). United European Gastroenterol J 2018;6(4):531; with permission.)

diagnostic endoscopy performed in the operating room or outpatient endoscopy center.[58] Saeian and colleagues[59] reported that there is no significant difference in detecting BE and dysplasia between unsedated transnasal endoscopy and conventional sedated endoscopy. This finding has been further confirmed by a randomized, blinded cross-over study that involved 121 patients who underwent sequential standard endoscopy followed by transnasal endoscopy or transnasal endoscopy followed by standard endoscopy for either GERD symptoms or surveillance of BE. The prevalence of BE in the

conventional endoscopy group and the unsedated transnasal endoscopy group was comparable at 26% and 30%, respectively ($P = .503$).[60] Another randomized cross-over study comparing transnasal endoscopy and standard endoscopy demonstrated that there was no difference in the endoscopic detection of BE ($P = .89$) and overall sensitivity, and specificity for detecting BE were 98% and 100%, respectively.[61] Both randomized studies showed better overall acceptance and tolerance of transnasal endoscopy over standard endoscopy.[60,61] Shariff and colleagues[62] recently published a pilot study evaluating the efficacy of transnasal endosheath endoscopy over standard endoscopy for detecting BE and dysplasia. Transnasal endosheath endoscope (TNE-5000 with EndoSheath Technology, Vision Sciences, Incorporated, New York) has been designed to bypass the need for reprocessing, and to allow use in a portable office-based setting. The instrument consists of a reusable ultrathin endoscope with an outer disposable sterile sheath and briefcase-size portable processor with light source and screen. The randomized cross-over study with this device has not been conducted yet, although it remains promising.[62] Ultimately, the widespread use of transnasal endoscopy could reduce the cost and improve the availability of BE screening.

SUMMARY

The incidence of esophageal adenocarcinoma has been increasing rapidly in Western countries over the past 30 years. Even though the risk of developing esophageal cancer in the setting of BE is low, it is a common premalignant condition for dysplasia and adenocarcinoma.[2,63] Although the early detection of BE is important, the incident of esophageal adenocarcinoma is still relatively rare compared with other malignancies. As such, the screening for BE is not recommended in the general population currently. Surveillance of BE is recommended to detect dysplasia and neoplasia in the early stage, although there is no significant evidence that surveillance reduces overall mortality of esophageal adenocarcinoma. Upper endoscopy is the current standard diagnostic, screening, and surveillance modality. For screening BE, less-invasive and cost-effective methods including transnasal endoscopy and nonendoscopic sampling techniques have been investigated and show promising results but still need further evaluation to be validated. Endoscopic surveillance with the Seattle protocol is widely accepted as the standard method for surveillance in BE. To improve accuracy of surveillance in BE, advanced imaging techniques including chromoendoscopy and electronic chromoendoscopy with magnification/high-definition endoscopy enable targeted biopsies in combination with the Seattle protocol. A new tissue sampling technique (WATS[3D]) in combination with Seattle protocol appears promising to elevate the accuracy of surveillance in BE. Further investigations ultimately are needed to assess the efficacy and utility of the various aforementioned approaches to the screening and surveillance of BE.

REFERENCES

1. Cameron AJ. Epidemiology of columnar-lined esophagus and adenocarcinoma. Gastroenterol Clin North Am 1997;26(3):487–94.
2. Bennett C, Moayyedi P, Corley DA, et al. BOB CAT: a large-scale review and delphi consensus for management of barrett's esophagus with no dysplasia, indefinite for, or low-grade dysplasia. Am J Gastroenterol 2015;110(5):662–82 [quiz: 683].
3. Blot WJ. Esophageal cancer trends and risk factors. Semin Oncol 1994;21(4):403–10.
4. Daly JM, Karnell LH, Menck HR. National cancer data base report on esophageal carcinoma. Cancer 1996;78(8):1820–8.
5. Hesketh PJ, Clapp RW, Doos WG, et al. The increasing frequency of adenocarcinoma of the esophagus. Cancer 15 1989;64(2):526–30.
6. Cameron AJ, Ott BJ, Payne WS. The incidence of adenocarcinoma in columnar-lined (Barrett's) esophagus. N Engl J Med 1985;313(14):857–9.
7. Hvid-Jensen F, Pedersen L, Drewes AM, et al. Incidence of adenocarcinoma among patients with Barrett's esophagus. N Engl J Med 2011;365(15):1375–83.
8. Bhat S, Coleman HG, Yousef F, et al. Risk of malignant progression in Barrett's esophagus patients: results from a large population-based study. J Natl Cancer Inst 2011;103(13):1049–57.
9. Rex DK, Cummings OW, Shaw M, et al. Screening for Barrett's esophagus in colonoscopy patients with and without heartburn. Gastroenterology 2003;125(6):1670–7.
10. Ward EM, Wolfsen HC, Achem SR, et al. Barrett's esophagus is common in older men and women undergoing screening colonoscopy regardless of reflux symptoms. Am J Gastroenterol 2006;101(1):12–7.
11. Cook MB, Wild CP, Forman D. A systematic review and meta-analysis of the sex ratio for Barrett's esophagus, erosive reflux disease, and nonerosive reflux disease. Am J Epidemiol 2005;162(11):1050–61.
12. Conio M, Cameron AJ, Romero Y, et al. Secular trends in the epidemiology and outcome of Barrett's oesophagus in Olmsted County, Minnesota. Gut 2001;48(3):304–9.
13. Sharma P, Morales TG, Sampliner RE. Short segment Barrett's esophagus–the need for standardization of the definition and of endoscopic criteria. Am J Gastroenterol 1998;93(7):1033–6.
14. Thomas T, Abrams KR, De Caestecker JS, et al. Meta analysis: cancer risk in Barrett's oesophagus. Aliment Pharmacol Ther 2007;26(11–12):1465–77.
15. Sharma P, Dent J, Armstrong D, et al. The development and validation of an endoscopic grading system for Barrett's esophagus: the Prague C & M criteria. Gastroenterology 2006;131(5):1392–9.
16. Wang KK, Sampliner RE, Practice parameters Committee of the American College of Gastroenterology. Updated guidelines 2008 for the diagnosis, surveillance and therapy of Barrett's esophagus. Am J Gastroenterol 2008;103(3):788–97.
17. Sharma P. Clinical practice. Barrett's esophagus. N Engl J Med 2009;361(26):2548–56.
18. Cameron AJ, Carpenter HA. Barrett's esophagus, high-grade dysplasia, and early adenocarcinoma: a pathological study. Am J Gastroenterol 1997;92(4):586–91.
19. Falk GW, Rice TW, Goldblum JR, et al. Jumbo biopsy forceps protocol still misses unsuspected cancer in Barrett's esophagus with high-grade dysplasia. Gastrointest Endosc 1999;49(2):170–6.
20. Boerwinkel DF, Swager A, Curvers WL, et al. The clinical consequences of advanced imaging techniques in Barrett's esophagus. Gastroenterology 2014;146(3):622–9.e4.
21. Sharma P, McQuaid K, Dent J, et al. A critical review of the diagnosis and management of Barrett's esophagus: the AGA Chicago workshop. Gastroenterology 2004;127(1):310–30.
22. Levine DS, Blount PL, Rudolph RE, et al. Safety of a systematic endoscopic biopsy protocol in patients with Barrett's esophagus. Am J Gastroenterol 2000;95(5):1152–7.

23. Naveed M, Dunbar KB. Endoscopic imaging of Barrett's esophagus. World J Gastrointest Endosc 2016; 8(5):259–66.
24. Gill RS, Singh R. Endoscopic imaging in Barrett's esophagus: current practice and future applications. Ann Gastroenterol 2012;25(2):89–95.
25. Sharma P, Weston AP, Topalovski M, et al. Magnification chromoendoscopy for the detection of intestinal metaplasia and dysplasia in Barrett's oesophagus. Gut 2003;52(1):24–7.
26. Canto MI. Chromoendoscopy and magnifying endoscopy for Barrett's esophagus. Clin Gastroenterol Hepatol 2005;3(7 Suppl 1):S12–5.
27. Canto MI, Setrakian S, Willis J, et al. Methylene blue-directed biopsies improve detection of intestinal metaplasia and dysplasia in Barrett's esophagus. Gastrointest Endosc 2000;51(5):560–8.
28. Ngamruengphong S, Sharma VK, Das A. Diagnostic yield of methylene blue chromoendoscopy for detecting specialized intestinal metaplasia and dysplasia in Barrett's esophagus: a meta-analysis. Gastrointest Endosc 2009;69(6):1021–8.
29. Hoffman A, Kiesslich R, Bender A, et al. Acetic acid-guided biopsies after magnifying endoscopy compared with random biopsies in the detection of Barrett's esophagus: a prospective randomized trial with crossover design. Gastrointest Endosc 2006; 64(1):1–8.
30. Reaud S, Croue A, Boyer J. Diagnostic accuracy of magnifying chromoendoscopy with detection of intestinal metaplasia and dysplasia using acetic acid in Barrett's esophagus. Gastroenterol Clin Biol 2006;30(2):217–23.
31. Hoffman A, Korczynski O, Tresch A, et al. Acetic acid compared with i-scan imaging for detecting Barrett's esophagus: a randomized, comparative trial. Gastrointest Endosc 2014;79(1):46–54.
32. Kono Y, Takenaka R, Kawahara Y, et al. Chromoendoscopy of gastric adenoma using an acetic acid indigocarmine mixture. World J Gastroenterol 2014; 20(17):5092–7.
33. Coletta M, Sami SS, Nachiappan A, et al. Acetic acid chromoendoscopy for the diagnosis of early neoplasia and specialized intestinal metaplasia in Barrett's esophagus: a meta-analysis. Gastrointest Endosc 2016;83(1):57–67.e1.
34. Tholoor S, Bhattacharyya R, Tsagkournis O, et al. Acetic acid chromoendoscopy in Barrett's esophagus surveillance is superior to the standardized random biopsy protocol: results from a large cohort study (with video). Gastrointest Endosc 2014;80(3): 417–24.
35. Longcroft-Wheaton G, Duku M, Mead R, et al. Acetic acid spray is an effective tool for the endoscopic detection of neoplasia in patients with Barrett's esophagus. Clin Gastroenterol Hepatol 2010;8(10): 843–7.
36. Bhandari P, Kandaswamy P, Cowlishaw D, et al. Acetic acid-enhanced chromoendoscopy is more cost-effective than protocol-guided biopsies in a high-risk Barrett's population. Dis Esophagus 2012; 25(5):386–92.
37. Committee AT, Manfredi MA, Abu Dayyeh BK, et al. Electronic chromoendoscopy. Gastrointest Endosc 2015;81(2):249–61.
38. Gono K, Obi T, Yamaguchi M, et al. Appearance of enhanced tissue features in narrow-band endoscopic imaging. J Biomed Opt 2004;9(3):568–77.
39. Kuznetsov K, Lambert R, Rey JF. Narrow-band imaging: potential and limitations. Endoscopy 2006; 38(1):76–81.
40. Sharma P. Narrow band imaging in Barrett's esophagus. Clin Gastroenterol Hepatol 2005;3(7 Suppl 1): S21–2.
41. Goda K, Tajiri H, Ikegami M, et al. Usefulness of magnifying endoscopy with narrow band imaging for the detection of specialized intestinal metaplasia in columnar-lined esophagus and Barrett's adenocarcinoma. Gastrointest Endosc 2007;65(1): 36–46.
42. Sharma P, Hawes RH, Bansal A, et al. Standard endoscopy with random biopsies versus narrow band imaging targeted biopsies in Barrett's oesophagus: a prospective, international, randomised controlled trial. Gut 2013;62(1):15–21.
43. Kara MA, Ennahachi M, Fockens P, et al. Detection and classification of the mucosal and vascular patterns (mucosal morphology) in Barrett's esophagus by using narrow band imaging. Gastrointest Endosc 2006;64(2):155–66.
44. Sharma P, Bansal A, Mathur S, et al. The utility of a novel narrow band imaging endoscopy system in patients with Barrett's esophagus. Gastrointest Endosc 2006;64(2):167–75.
45. Anagnostopoulos GK, Yao K, Kaye P, et al. Novel endoscopic observation in Barrett's oesophagus using high resolution magnification endoscopy and narrow band imaging. Aliment Pharmacol Ther 2007;26(3):501–7.
46. Singh R, Anagnostopoulos GK, Yao K, et al. Narrow-band imaging with magnification in Barrett's esophagus: validation of a simplified grading system of mucosal morphology patterns against histology. Endoscopy 2008;40(6):457–63.
47. Singh M, Bansal A, Curvers WL, et al. Observer agreement in the assessment of narrowband imaging system surface patterns in Barrett's esophagus: a multicenter study. Endoscopy 2011;43(9):745–51.
48. Silva FB, Dinis-Ribeiro M, Vieth M, et al. Endoscopic assessment and grading of Barrett's esophagus using magnification endoscopy and narrow-band imaging: accuracy and interobserver agreement of different classification systems (with videos). Gastrointest Endosc 2011;73(1):7–14.

49. Curvers WL, Bohmer CJ, Mallant-Hent RC, et al. Mucosal morphology in Barrett's esophagus: inter-observer agreement and role of narrow band imaging. Endoscopy 2008;40(10):799–805.

50. Curvers W, Baak L, Kiesslich R, et al. Chromoendoscopy and narrow-band imaging compared with high-resolution magnification endoscopy in Barrett's esophagus. Gastroenterology 2008;134(3):670–9.

51. Sharma P, Bergman JJ, Goda K, et al. Development and validation of a classification system to identify high-grade dysplasia and esophageal adenocarcinoma in barrett's esophagus using narrow-band imaging. Gastroenterology 2016;150(3):591–8.

52. Vennalaganti PR, Kaul V, Wang KK, et al. Increased detection of Barrett's esophagus-associated neoplasia using wide-area trans-epithelial sampling: a multicenter, prospective, randomized trial. Gastrointest Endosc 2018;87(2):348–55.

53. Gross SA, Smith MS, Kaul V, et al. Increased detection of Barrett's esophagus and esophageal dysplasia with adjunctive use of wide-area transepithelial sample with three-dimensional computer-assisted analysis (WATS). United European Gastroenterol J 2018;6(4):529–35.

54. Lao-Sirieix P, Boussioutas A, Kadri SR, et al. Non-endoscopic screening biomarkers for Barrett's oesophagus: from microarray analysis to the clinic. Gut 2009;58(11):1451–9.

55. Kadri SR, Lao-Sirieix P, O'Donovan M, et al. Acceptability and accuracy of a non-endoscopic screening test for Barrett's oesophagus in primary care: cohort study. BMJ 2010;341:c4372.

56. Ross-Innes CS, Debiram-Beecham I, O'Donovan M, et al. Evaluation of a minimally invasive cell sampling device coupled with assessment of trefoil factor 3 expression for diagnosing Barrett's esophagus: a multi-center case-control study. PLoS Med 2015; 12(1):e1001780.

57. Benaglia T, Sharples LD, Fitzgerald RC, et al. Health benefits and cost effectiveness of endoscopic and nonendoscopic cytosponge screening for Barrett's esophagus. Gastroenterology 2013; 144(1):62–73.e6.

58. Saeian K. Unsedated transnasal endoscopy: a safe and less costly alternative. Curr Gastroenterol Rep 2002;4(3):213–7.

59. Saeian K, Staff DM, Vasilopoulos S, et al. Unsedated transnasal endoscopy accurately detects Barrett's metaplasia and dysplasia. Gastrointest Endosc 2002;56(4):472–8.

60. Jobe BA, Hunter JG, Chang EY, et al. Office-based unsedated small-caliber endoscopy is equivalent to conventional sedated endoscopy in screening and surveillance for Barrett's esophagus: a randomized and blinded comparison. Am J Gastroenterol 2006;101(12):2693–703.

61. Shariff MK, Bird-Lieberman EL, O'Donovan M, et al. Randomized crossover study comparing efficacy of transnasal endoscopy with that of standard endoscopy to detect Barrett's esophagus. Gastrointest Endosc 2012;75(5):954–61.

62. Shariff MK, Varghese S, O'Donovan M, et al. Pilot randomized crossover study comparing the efficacy of transnasal disposable endosheath with standard endoscopy to detect Barrett's esophagus. Endoscopy 2016;48(2):110–6.

63. Fitzgerald RC, di Pietro M, Ragunath K, et al. British Society of Gastroenterology guidelines on the diagnosis and management of Barrett's oesophagus. Gut 2014;63(1):7–42.

Advanced Endoluminal Technologies for Barrett's Esophagus
Focus on Optical Coherence Tomography and Confocal Laser Endomicroscopy

Ahmed M. Zihni, MD, MPH[a,b,c],
Steven R. DeMeester, MD[a,c],*

KEYWORDS

- Barrett's esophagus • Endomicroscopy • Optical coherence tomography

KEY POINTS

- Barrett's esophagus is a premalignant condition of the esophagus characterized by replacement of the normal squamous mucosa with intestinal metaplasia.
- Detection of dysplasia indicates progression of disease.
- New imaging technologies allow real-time evaluation of the Barrett's mucosa for disease progression.

INTRODUCTION

High-definition flexible endoscopes allow detailed evaluation of the esophageal mucosa and identification of the squamocolumnar junction, as well as islands, tongues, or a circumferential extension of columnar mucosa into the esophagus. These extensions of columnar mucosa may have only columnar cells, called cardiac mucosa, or may have goblet cells, which indicate intestinal metaplasia. Intestinal metaplasia, the hallmark of Barrett's esophagus (BE), is a premalignant, metaplastic transformation of normal squamous mucosa induced by damage from the reflux of gastric juice into the esophagus. Once it has developed, BE may progress to dysplasia and, ultimately, adenocarcinoma.

Most high-definition upper endoscopes allow evaluation of the mucosa with narrow-band imaging (NBI) or a similar feature that further accentuates columnar mucosa and allows better evaluation of BE. However, neither high-definition white light nor NBI will allow reliable determination of the presence of intestinal metaplasia or dysplasia within a columnar segment of mucosa. Until recently, this required biopsies and histologic evaluation of the tissue by a pathologist using a microscope. Further, in the absence of irregular features in the columnar mucosa, such as nodules or ulcers, these biopsies are obtained in a random fashion from the columnar mucosa. The problems with this approach are that these random biopsies may miss areas of dysplasia or early adenocarcinoma, and that the biopsies take several days to process and be read by the pathologist, so findings are not available in real time during the upper endoscopy. Two important technologies are available to facilitate the detection of Barrett's and

---

[a] Division of Gastrointestinal and Minimally Invasive Surgery, The Oregon Clinic, 4805 NE Glisan Street, Suite 6N60, Portland, OR 97213, USA; [b] Providence Portland Medical Center, 4805 NE Glisan Street, Suite 6N60, Portland, OR 97213, USA; [c] The Foundation for Surgical Innovation and Education, 4805 NE Glisan Street, Suite 6N60, Portland, OR 97213, USA
* Corresponding author. The Oregon Clinic, 4805 NE Glisan Street, Suite 6N60, Portland, OR 97213.
E-mail address: sdemeester@orclinic.com

dysplasia in real time and overcome the limitations of random surveillance endoscopy. Further, they may have the utility to predict response to ablation and detect residual disease after ablation therapy. These technologies are probe-based confocal laser endomicroscopy (pCLE) and volumetric laser endomicroscopy (VLE) based on optical coherence tomography (OCT). Each of these is discussed in detail.

PROBE-BASED CONFOCAL LASER ENDOMICROSCOPY

Cellvizio (Mauna Kea Technologies, Paris, France) took the concepts of confocal endomicroscopy and extended the capabilities, allowing it to be used via probes passed down the working channel of an endoscope; thereby extending the capabilities of a high-definition flexible endoscope to allow real-time assessment of cellular and subcellular architecture within tissue. Traditional microscopes are wide-field microscopes in which the entire sample volume is illuminated at the same time. Confocal microscopy was patented in 1957 and, in contrast to conventional microscopes, confocal microscopes focus a beam of light into a small area inside tissue. The same objective that delivered the light gathers the reflected light and sends it through a pinhole aperture that allows only the light emitted from the desired focal spot to pass through to the detector. Scattered light that would degrade the image is thereby blocked. The pinhole is placed in a conjugate focal plane to the tissue specimen, hence the designation confocal.[1] Further, instead of the image going to the human eye, it is relayed to a light-sensitive detector where the incident photons are converted into an electrical signal that can be amplified by many orders of magnitude.[2] Confocal microscopy built on the advances of immunofluorescence microscopy but the practical applications of confocal microscopy for biological fluorescence imaging really became possible with the introduction of the first laser scanning confocal microscopes in 1987.[3] These systems rapidly and serially scan the focal spot and yield horizontal virtual-sectioned images that are recorded by a computer, which reconstructs the images 1 pixel at a time.

Cellvizio uses these confocal concepts to capture microscopic images of tissue in vivo. Laser light of a defined wavelength is passed down proprietary miniprobes that contain thousands of optical fibers. These probes are small enough to go down the working channel of an endoscope, whereas the laser scanning unit and the light source remain outside the body. Cellvizio uses specialized software to collect, stabilize, and display images to the detail of blood on a single erythrocyte scale in real time during the procedure. Imaging is optimized for deep observation of the mucosa, up to 150 microns, which is ideal for assessing premalignant and malignant changes. Cellvizio is used in combination with a contrast agent. Intravenous fluorescein is the current contrast agent of choice because it is relatively inexpensive, nonmutagenic, enables higher imaging depth than topically administered contrast agents, and has been safely used for decades in ophthalmology. Optimal contrast is obtained within the first 10 minutes after injection; however, good quality images can be acquired for a further 30 to 60 minutes.[4]

Performing the procedure is straightforward. After the esophagus has been examined with white light and NBI, and any areas of concern identified, intravenous fluorescein dye is given and a dissecting cap attached to the end of the endoscope. The cap helps stabilize the mucosa during imaging. The endoscope is reinserted into the esophagus and the Cellvizio miniprobe advanced down the biopsy channel. The tip of the probe is placed on the mucosa and the tissue examined. Because blood and mucus will degrade the image quality, it is best to avoid any biopsies and irrigate any mucus or debris out of the esophagus before imaging. Whenever possible, the probe should be oriented perpendicular to the mucosa for best image quality. Applying slight suction can help pull mucosa into the cap and hold the probe in a good position for imaging. The senior author (SRD) tends to start distally near the gastroesophageal junction (GEJ) and identify gastric mucosa to confirm the location of the GEJ. Then I image any irregular areas within the columnar-lined esophagus and randomly, with particular attention near the squamocolumnar junction, looking for evidence of goblet cells. These optical biopsies are then supplemented with targeted or routine biopsies or the wide-area transepithelial sampling (WATS) brush (CDx Diagnostics [Suffern, NY]).

The Cellvizio system allows for identification of foregut mucosa, including normal oxyntic mucosa, antral mucosa, gastric intestinal metaplasia, squamous mucosa, cardiac mucosa, cardiac mucosa with intestinal metaplasia (BE), dysplasia, and adenocarcinoma. The Miami classification provides useful descriptors for Barrett's, dysplasia, and adenocarcinoma.[4] On pCLE, the normal oxyntic gastric mucosa is characterized by dark, donut-shaped circles, the gastric glands (**Fig. 1**). Cardiac columnar mucosa shows a uniform villiform architecture and columnar cells without goblet cells (**Fig. 2**), whereas the addition of dark

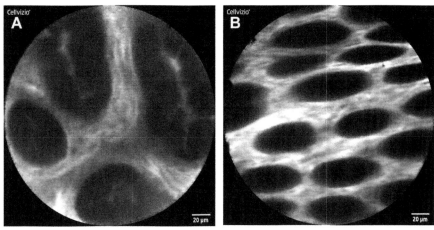

Fig. 1. (*A*) Oxyntic gastric mucosa is recognized by the presence of gastric pits that appear as round, regularly shaped dark circles. (*B*) Note the well-organized pattern. (*Courtesy of* Mauna Kea Technologies, Paris, France; with permission.)

round goblet cells to cardiac columnar mucosa defines intestinal metaplasia (**Fig. 3**). Dysplasia within columnar mucosa shows a villiform structure with dark, irregularly thickened epithelial borders and dilated irregular vessels (**Fig. 4**). Esophageal adenocarcinoma (EAC) is recognized by a disorganized or absent villiform structure, multiple dark columnar cells, and dilated irregular vessels (**Fig. 5**). Squamous mucosa has a fish-scale appearance, with flat cells without crypts or villi, and bright vessels found within the papillae (**Fig. 6**).

An early study with Cellvizio in subjects with dysplasia showed that the accuracy was 82% with a positive predictive value of 76% and a negative predictive value of 85%. Interobserver agreement on the diagnosis was substantial (kappa 0.61). When the images were judged to be of good quality, both the accuracy and agreement increased (95%; kappa 0.89). Further, when the reviewers were confident about their assessment of the images, the accuracy (98%) and agreement (kappa 0 .95) were excellent. The investigators also noted that there was a short learning curve for interpretation of the images.[5]

In clinical practice, an international, multicenter, prospective, randomized controlled trial showed that the addition of pCLE to high-definition endoscopy with or without NBI for evaluation of BE significantly improved the ability to detect

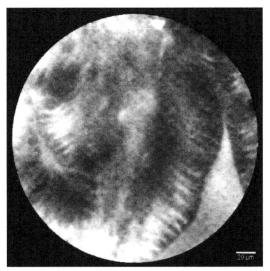

Fig. 2. Cardiac mucosa appears as a columnar epithelium with regularly spaced glands and cells. Dark goblet cells are absent.

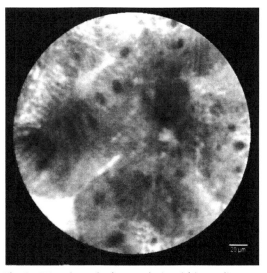

Fig. 3. BE, or intestinal metaplasia within cardiac mucosa, is similar to cardiac mucosa with the addition of dark round goblet cells. The glands are regular and nicely organized.

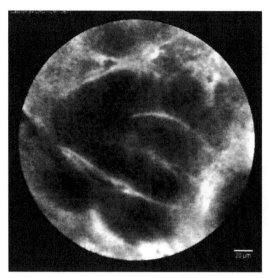

Fig. 4. Dysplasia within Barrett's is characterized by several features, including dark, irregular, disorganized glands and the absence of obvious goblet cells.

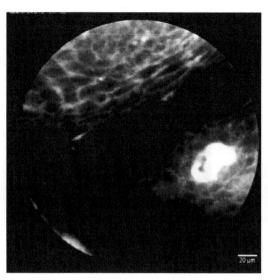

Fig. 6. Squamous mucosa is recognized as light gray, flat, scale-like cells. An intrapapillary loop may also be present as seen in the bottom right corner.

neoplasia. They reported that pCLE detected an additional 41 areas of high-grade dysplasia (HGD)-EAC in 122 subjects when lesions visible by high-definition endoscopy were excluded. The investigators concluded that if targeted and random biopsies were only performed in patients with suspicious lesions by endoscopy with NBI and pCLE, 39% of patients could forego biopsies and no one with HGD-EAC would have been missed.[6]

In a more recent retrospective study, pCLE correctly identified all cases of EAC in 55 subjects. One subject with short-segment Barrett's was

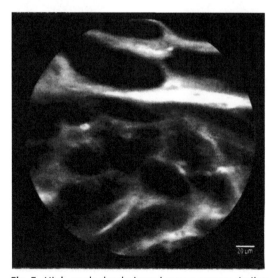

Fig. 5. High-grade dysplasia and cancer appear similar but with even more disorganized glands and pleomorphic enlarged cells.

considered to have nondysplastic BE by pCLE but random biopsies and subsequent endoscopic resection confirmed HGD. Overall, pCLE had a sensitivity of 67%, specificity of 98%, and positive predictive value of 67% for detection of HGD-EAC. Sensitivity of pCLE for low-grade dysplasia (LGD) was low compared with random biopsies. The investigators concluded that pCLE showed a high specificity for dysplasia and cancer, and affirmed the use of pCLE for real-time confirmation of a diagnosis of LGD in patients with Barrett's. However, they suggested that the relative lack of sensitivity and the lack of an incremental benefit over high-definition endoscopy with NBI might limit its utility in routine BE surveillance.[7]

In another study, pCLE was compared with Seattle protocol and targeted biopsies in subjects with at least LGD. The gold standard was pathologic assessment of the endoscopically resected area (either endoscopic mucosal resection or endoscopic submucosal dissection of the imaged area). There were 35 endoscopic resections in 31 subjects. A correct diagnosis was made in 71% (25 out of 35) of the cases by pCLE and in 43% (15 out of 35) of the cases by preresection biopsy. The sensitivity, specificity, and accuracy for the detection of HGD-EAC were 92.9%, 71.4%, and 80% for pCLE, respectively, and 78.6%, 61.9%, and 68.6% for histologic biopsy, respectively. However, the differences in favor of pCLE were not statistically significant ($P = .25$). One case of HGD-EAC was missed by pCLE and 3 cases were missed by the preresection biopsies. Thirteen subjects exhibited irregularities of the mucosa without elevated or depressed lesions (2

HGD-EAC cases and 11 non–HGD-EAC cases). Among these 13 subjects, pCLE led to positive re-directions of therapy in 70% (9 out of 13) of the cases. There was one misdiagnosis (8%) but no cases of HGD-EAC were missed by pCLE. In these cases, pCLE exhibited a sensitivity, specificity, and accuracy for the detection of HGD-EAC of 100%, 82%, and 85%, respectively, compared with 55%, 50%, and 54%, respectively, for the preresection biopsies ($P = .22$). The investigators concluded that pCLE could aid in management and decision-making in patients with dysplastic BE before endoscopic therapy, particularly in the absence of a visible lesion in the mucosa.[8]

Finally, a meta-analysis was performed of the columnar-lined esophagus for detection of dysplasia in BE. The analysis, including 14 studies, 789 subjects, and 4047 lesions, reported that the pooled sensitivity and specificity for the per-subject analysis were 89% (95% CI 0.82–0.94) and 83% (95% CI 0.78–0.86), respectively. When a per-lesion analysis was performed, the corre-sponding pooled sensitivity declined to 77% (95% CI 0.73–0.81) and specificity increased to 89% (95% CI 0.87–0.90). The investigators concluded that pCLE can accurately differentiate neoplasms from nonneoplasms in patients with BE, using histopathology as the reference stan-dard. Further, they suggested that pCLE is a valid, in vivo, real-time noninvasive method for surveil-lance and early diagnosis of esophageal neo-plasms in patients with BE.[9]

Cellvizio is not limited to the esophageal mu-cosa but has been found useful for evaluation of the biliary tree, pancreatic cysts, and the colon, among other sites. In addition, it has been used to evaluate the esophageal myenteric plexus in patients with achalasia undergoing peroral endo-scopic myotomy, and to evaluate resection mar-gins in patients having endoscopic resections or endoscopic submucosal dissections for esopha-geal or gastric malignancies. This technology has broad applicability, provides cellular-level imaging in real time, and will continue to serve important roles in the management of patients with condi-tions that can be reached with an endoscope.

OPTICAL COHERENCE TOMOGRAPHY AND VOLUMETRIC LASER ENDOMICROSCOPY

OCT is a form of optical ultrasonography in which reflected light waves, instead of sound waves, are used to obtain subsurface, cross-sectional images of a mucosal surface. The working principle of OCT is based on an optical ranging technique known as low-coherence interferometry, whereby the time delay and signal intensity of light reflected

back from a sample is measured. The images ob-tained are many times higher resolution than those obtained using high-frequency ultrasound, and are able to show mucosal and submucosal structures in microscopic detail. This level of detail comes at the price of limited depth of imaging.[10] NvisionVLE (NinePoint Medical, Inc, Bedford, MA, USA) is a second-generation OCT technology that uses infrared light to produce real-time, high-resolution, cross-sectional, microstructure imaging of tissue. The components of the system are a console, monitor, and balloon-based probes that attach to the console. The balloon centers the probe in the lumen of the esophagus and distends the esoph-agus to minimize folds in the tissue to be imaged. Imaging is performed by automatic helical pullback of the probe from the distal to the proximal end of the balloon. This system scans a 6-cm length of the tubular esophagus in approximately 90 seconds and produce images with an axial resolution of 7 mm to a depth up to 3 mm.[10] One scan produces approximately 1200 cross-sectional images that are viewed by using a software interface that allows simultaneous examination of cross-sectional, transverse, and longitudinal views. A recent up-grade to the system includes a positional controller that is attached to the body of the endoscope (just below the biopsy channel inlet). The controller has several functions, including manual control of the VLE scan, image capture, and tags for regions of in-terest. Further, this upgrade allows the option of su-perficial, cautery-type laser markings of a region of interest for subsequent biopsy or endoscopic resection. The endoscopist can select either a sin-gle mark or double laser marks spaced approxi-mately 1 cm apart to more precisely localize an abnormal area on or below the mucosa.[11]

The NinePoint VLE system is easy to use. After evaluation of the esophagus with a high-definition upper endoscope with NBI, the VLE balloon is positioned across the GEJ, inflated, and the scan obtained. Immediate review of the images allows identification of any areas of concern. The normal squamous mucosa with typical layering pattern is easy to recognize (**Fig. 7**), as is columnar mucosa with loss of layer-ing (**Fig. 8**). Detection of mucosal changes, such as dysplasia or cancer, is more challenging (**Fig. 9**). Likewise, although recognition of subsur-face glands is not difficult, discerning whether they are normal structures or an abnormal area of concern involves a learning curve. A recent study evaluated the learning curve for VLE. A group of 31 novice VLE physicians underwent brief online training and then were asked to evaluate a set of 24 VLE images of each of 4 types of mu-cosa. The VLE images were from normal gastric

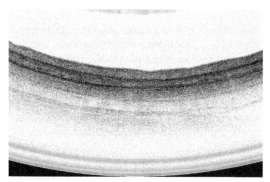

Fig. 7. Squamous mucosa on OCT is recognized by uniform layering of the esophageal wall showing the mucosa, submucosa, and 2 layers of the muscularis propria moving from the lumen outward. (*Courtesy of* Nine-Point Medical, Inc, Bedford, MA; with permission).

cardia, normal esophageal squamous epithelium, nonneoplastic BE, and neoplastic BE. The average time to complete the training session was 59 minutes. A total of 22 physicians (71%) achieved competency (defined as a failure rate of <10%) during the study. The median accuracy for esophageal squamous epithelium, gastric epithelium, nonneoplastic BE, and neoplastic BE was 96%, 95%, 90%, and 96%, respectively. Although most users achieved competence, there was a high degree of variability with regard to number of images reviewed to reach competence, although all were within the range of a short 1-hour to 2-hour training and testing session. The investigators concluded that, similar to other advanced imaging technologies, there is a rapid learning curve and competence can be achieved by most novice VLE users after a computer training session.[12]

In clinical practice, VLE has been used to screen for BE, for surveillance of known Barrett's for evidence of dysplasia, and for mapping of dysplastic Barrett's before ablation or endoscopic resection. In these areas, VLE competes with other technologies. However, an important niche for VLE is in the follow-up of patients after endoscopic resection or ablation therapy. No other technology allows imaging below the neosquamous mucosa to detect buried or residual Barrett's glands. In a study of 17 subjects who had been endoscopically treated to no visible Barrett's mucosa, high-definition endoscopy showed no lesions or areas of abnormality. However, VLE showed 1 or more areas of subsquamous glandular structure (SGS) in 13 (76%) of the subjects. The frequency of finding buried Barrett's in an area of SGS was 8%.[13] Although often these SGS are benign, detection of buried cancer has been reported and the use of VLE likely prevented a more advanced cancer from developing.[14] Recently, laser marking capabilities have been added to VLE that allow marking of areas of concern for subsequent resection. An early study using the laser marking technology showed that all of the laser marks were endoscopically visible in the Barrett's mucosa, and all of the suspicious regions noted by VLE were successfully laser marked for endoscopic resection or biopsy.[15]

An interesting potential use for VLE is to predict the efficacy of ablation therapy based on the pretreatment thickness of the metaplastic or dysplastic mucosa. A study using endoscopic OCT showed that, compared with subjects with thinner Barrett's, those with a Barrett's mucosal thickness of greater than 333 microns were more likely to have OCT-detected residual glands immediately after radiofrequency ablation, as well as persistent areas of Barrett's on endoscopic follow-up 6 to 8 weeks postablation. The

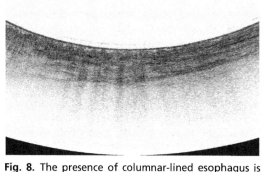

Fig. 8. The presence of columnar-lined esophagus is indicated on OCT by loss of the normal layering pattern. Here, the esophageal wall is recognized but the mucosa, submucosa, and muscularis propria layers are indistinct. (*Courtesy of* NinePoint Medical, Inc, Bedford, MA; with permission).

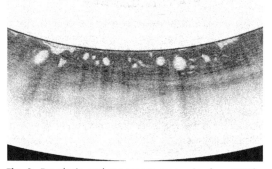

Fig. 9. Dysplasia and cancer are recognized on OCT by a dark appearance to the superficial layers and glandular structures in the subsurface layers. (*Courtesy of* NinePoint Medical, Inc, Bedford, MA; with permission).

investigators noted that OCT could identify residual glands despite the debris and mucosal sluff caused by the ablation. They concluded that the presence of thicker Barrett's mucosa suggests the need for more aggressive ablation, whereas the presence of residual glands immediately after ablation suggests the need for additional ablation.[16]

A promising area for VLE is in dysplasia and cancer detection during endoscopic Barrett's surveillance. In a retrospective series of 386 subjects with BE and no visible lesion, VLE with laser marking significantly increased the rate of dysplasia detection compared with either random biopsies or Seattle protocol biopsies.[17] Features in BE that on VLE are associated with dysplasia and cancer include a darker appearance of the surface compared with the deeper tissue (higher surface-to-subsurface intensity ratio); loss of horizontal layering; and the presence of irregular, dilated glands or ducts.[18] These features have been used to develop a diagnostic algorithm for dysplasia. The reported sensitivity, specificity, and diagnostic accuracy for the detection of dysplasia with the algorithm was 86%, 88%, and 87%, respectively, with almost perfect interobserver agreement (kappa 0.86).[11] Subsequently, a VLE neoplasia prediction score was developed that uses these features to assign points, with 8 or more points associated with an increased likelihood of neoplasia.[18,19] Often these changes, particularly the surface-to-subsurface intensity ratio, are subtle and potentially missed. Consequently, the future of VLE likely will entail computer-assisted analysis. Recently, a computer algorithm based on clinically derived features was shown to outperform a group of VLE experts for identification of early Barrett's neoplasia.[20] A logical extension of this technology is to have computer-aided real time analysis of VLE scans during BE surveillance with laser marking of suspicious areas for targeted biopsies or endoscopic resection. This promising technology may improve the outcomes with Barrett's surveillance.

Finally, OCT technology may offer the potential for BE screening in the form of a tethered, swallowed capsule. The capsule is approximately 12 mm in diameter and enables high-resolution circumferential OCT imaging of the esophagus. It does not require sedation or anesthesia, and an early clinical study demonstrated feasibility, high patient acceptability, and strong potential for clinical impact.[21] Following this feasibility study, the OCT capsule is now being used in a primary care setting for BE screening.[22] Subsequent modifications to the design of the capsule enabled precise rotary and longitudinal scanning that produces high-quality volumetric imaging with en face visualization and reduced motion-induced distortion.[23] If proven cost-effective, reliable, and well-tolerated, this capsule OCT technology could be used for screening of populations at risk for having BE.

SUMMARY

These technologies, pCLE and VLE, allow a detailed evaluation of the esophageal mucosa and submucosal structures in situ and in real time. Never before has so much detail been so easily obtained in patients with BE, dysplasia, or early adenocarcinoma. Like most technologies, early experience has been at centers with a defined interest in these conditions; however, as the methodology and capabilities get better clarified, it is likely that both of these devices will become essential tools at centers following patients with BE and performing endoscopic therapy for dysplastic Barrett's or early cancer.

REFERENCES

1. Nwaneshiudu A, Kuschal C, Sakamoto FH, et al. Introduction to confocal microscopy. J Invest Dermatol 2012;132:e3.
2. Vangindertael J, Camacho R, Sempels W, et al. An introduction to optical super-resolution microscopy for the adventurous biologist. Methods Appl Fluoresc 2018;6:022003.
3. Wallace MB. Somewhere over the rainbow. Gastrointest Endosc 2010;71:354–6.
4. Wallace M, Lauwers GY, Chen Y, et al. Miami classification for probe-based confocal laser endomicroscopy. Endoscopy 2011;43:882–91.
5. Tofteland N, Singh M, Gaddam S, et al. Evaluation of the updated confocal laser endomicroscopy criteria for Barrett's esophagus among gastrointestinal pathologists. Dis Esophagus 2014;27:623–9.
6. Sharma P, Meining AR, Coron E, et al. Real-time increased detection of neoplastic tissue in Barrett's esophagus with probe-based confocal laser endomicroscopy: final results of an international multicenter, prospective, randomized, controlled trial. Gastrointest Endosc 2011;74:465–72.
7. Shah T, Lippman R, Kohli D, et al. Accuracy of probe-based confocal laser endomicroscopy (pCLE) compared to random biopsies during endoscopic surveillance of Barrett's esophagus. Endosc Int open 2018;6:E414–20.
8. Caillol F, Godat S, Poizat F, et al. Probe confocal laser endomicroscopy in the therapeutic endoscopic management of Barrett's dysplasia. Ann Gastroenterol 2017;30:295–301.
9. Xiong YQ, Ma SJ, Zhou JH, et al. A meta-analysis of confocal laser endomicroscopy for the detection of

neoplasia in patients with Barrett's esophagus. J Gastroenterol Hepatol 2016;31:1102–10.

10. Tsai TH, Leggett CL, Trindade AJ, et al. Optical coherence tomography in gastroenterology: a review and future outlook. J Biomed Opt 2017;22: 1–17.

11. Leggett CL, Gorospe EC, Chan DK, et al. Comparative diagnostic performance of volumetric laser endomicroscopy and confocal laser endomicroscopy in the detection of dysplasia associated with Barrett's esophagus. Gastrointest Endosc 2016;83: 880–8.e2.

12. Trindade AJ, Inamdar S, Smith MS, et al. Learning curve and competence for volumetric laser endomicroscopy in Barrett's esophagus using cumulative sum analysis. Endoscopy 2018;50:471–8.

13. Swager AF, Boerwinkel DF, de Bruin DM, et al. Detection of buried Barrett's glands after radiofrequency ablation with volumetric laser endomicroscopy. Gastrointest Endosc 2016;83:80–8.

14. Leggett CL, Gorospe E, Owens VL, et al. Volumetric laser endomicroscopy detects subsquamous Barrett's adenocarcinoma. Am J Gastroenterol 2014; 109:298–9.

15. Swager AF, de Groof AJ, Meijer SL, et al. Feasibility of laser marking in Barrett's esophagus with volumetric laser endomicroscopy: first-in-man pilot study. Gastrointest Endosc 2017;86: 464–72.

16. Tsai TH, Zhou C, Tao YK, et al. Structural markers observed with endoscopic 3-dimensional optical coherence tomography correlating with Barrett's esophagus radiofrequency ablation treatment response (with videos). Gastrointest Endosc 2012; 76:1104–12.

17. Alshelleh M, Inamdar S, McKinley M, et al. Incremental yield of dysplasia detection in Barrett's esophagus using volumetric laser endomicroscopy with and without laser marking compared with a standardized random biopsy protocol. Gastrointest Endosc 2018;88(1):35–42.

18. Swager AF, Tearney GJ, Leggett CL, et al. Identification of volumetric laser endomicroscopy features predictive for early neoplasia in Barrett's esophagus using high-quality histological correlation. Gastrointest Endosc 2017;85:918–26.e7.

19. van der Sommen F, Klomp SR, Swager AF, et al. Predictive features for early cancer detection in Barrett's esophagus using Volumetric Laser Endomicroscopy. Comput Med Imaging Graph 2018;67:9–20.

20. Swager AF, van der Sommen F, Klomp SR, et al. Computer-aided detection of early Barrett's neoplasia using volumetric laser endomicroscopy. Gastrointest Endosc 2017;86:839–46.

21. Gora MJ, Sauk JS, Carruth RW, et al. Imaging the upper gastrointestinal tract in unsedated patients using tethered capsule endomicroscopy. Gastroenterology 2013;145:723–5.

22. Gora MJ, Simmons LH, Queneherve L, et al. Tethered capsule endomicroscopy: from bench to bedside at a primary care practice. J Biomed Opt 2016;21:104001.

23. Liang K, Ahsen OO, Lee HC, et al. Volumetric mapping of Barrett's esophagus and dysplasia with en face optical coherence tomography tethered capsule. Am J Gastroenterol 2016;111:1664–6.

Mucosal Ablation Techniques for Barrett's Esophagus and Early Esophageal Cancer

Ravi Rajaram, MD, MSc*, Wayne L. Hofstetter, MD

KEYWORDS

- Barrett's esophagus • Cryotherapy • Catheter ablation • Endoscopy • Esophageal neoplasm
- Esophagoscopy • Metaplasia • Precancerous conditions

KEY POINTS

- Barrett's esophagus is intestinal metaplasia of the normally squamous lined esophageal mucosa and can pathologically be classified as nondysplastic, low-grade dysplasia, or high-grade dysplasia.
- Radiofrequency ablation of Barrett's esophagus results in a high rate of eradication of intestinal metaplasia and dysplasia and a reduced risk of disease progression.
- Several studies have also reported high eradication rates of nondysplastic and dysplastic Barrett's esophagus with cryoablation, using both liquid nitrogen and pressurized carbon dioxide.
- Current guidelines support the use of ablation in patients with Barrett's esophagus with high-grade and low-grade dysplasia, although patients without dysplasia should undergo surveillance rather than ablation.

INTRODUCTION

Columnar-lined intestinal metaplasia of the normally squamous esophageal mucosa is termed Barrett's esophagus (BE). Gastroesophageal reflux disease (GERD) is considered one of the major risk factors for the development of BE, particularly in older patients with long-standing disease.[1] The estimated prevalence of GERD (19.8%) and BE (5.6%) have increased significantly in the United States in recent years, possibly related to increasing obesity rates.[2,3]

Endoscopically, BE characteristically appears as coarse salmon-colored mucosa in contrast to the pale or pearly colored stratified squamous epithelium that normally lines the inner esophagus.[4] Use of high-definition white light imaging or new imaging modalities including narrow band imaging, chromoendoscopy, optical coherence tomography, and laser confocal microscopy may improve the ability of endoscopists to detect BE, as well as any associated dysplastic changes.[4] A detailed review of these advanced endoluminal technologies is included elsewhere in this issue. In addition to its appearance, a diagnosis of BE is confirmed with biopsies demonstrating intestinal metaplasia ≥1 cm above the gastroesophageal junction.[5]

BE is further characterized as short-segment (<3 cm) or long-segment (≥3 cm). Additionally, the Prague Criteria is a classification system often used to describe the circumferential and maximal extent of metaplastic disease.[6] In addition to providing a common language among endoscopists to report the degree of BE present, this system

Disclosure Statement: The authors have nothing to disclose.
Department of Thoracic and Cardiovascular Surgery, The University of Texas MD Anderson Cancer Center, 1515 Holcombe Boulevard, Houston, TX 77030, USA
* Corresponding author.
E-mail address: rrajaram@mdanderson.org

Thorac Surg Clin 28 (2018) 473–480
https://doi.org/10.1016/j.thorsurg.2018.07.004

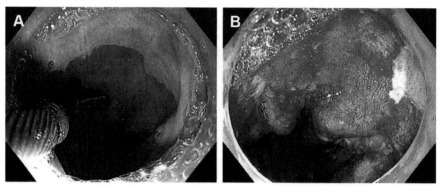

Fig. 1. RFA performed in a patient with BE. (*A*) Pre-ablation with catheter seen adjacent to area of metaplastic disease. (*B*) Posttreatment after RFA.

has also been prospectively validated as having a high reliability coefficient (RC) for recognizing BE segments ≥1 cm (RC 0.72), although not for segments <1 cm (RC 0.22).[6]

This use of endoscopic ablation therapies for the management of nondysplastic and dysplastic BE has grown considerably in the past several years. Although a number of different modalities have been described, including photodynamic therapy and argon plasma coagulation, they have largely been supplanted by evidence favoring the use of radiofrequency ablation (RFA). Additionally, several studies have demonstrated promising results from the use of cryoablation. This review highlights the use of RFA and cryoablation in BE and early esophageal adenocarcinoma (EAC), as well as current evidence-based guidelines for the use of these technologies.

RADIOFREQUENCY ABLATION

Endoscopic RFA is performed using a specialized heated ablation catheter for targeted, intentional mucosal injury and cellular destruction (**Fig. 1**). Energy conduction usually reaches the level of the lamina propria and is directed at areas of known or suspicious intestinal metaplasia and/or dysplasia. Several endoscopic treatment sessions are typically required to achieve complete eradication of intestinal metaplasia (CEIM). A successful outcome from endoscopic ablation is considered complete clearance of a patient's BE as well as any associated areas of dysplasia.[5] Evidence suggests that endoscopists with higher RFA volume may achieve higher rates of CEIM.[7]

Radiofrequency Ablation for Dysplastic Barrett's Esophagus

Several studies have evaluated the use of endoscopic RFA for the treatment of BE with or without dysplasia. The AIM Dysplasia Trial was a

multicenter study of patients with non-nodular dysplastic BE who were randomized to either RFA or a sham procedure.[8] Patients with both low-grade dysplasia (LGD) and high-grade dysplasia (HGD) were included. The primary outcomes of this study included the proportion of patients with CEIM by 12 months as well as eradication of both LGD and HGD during this period. In total, 127 patients were randomized. Intention-to-treat analyses demonstrated 77.4% of patients in the RFA group had CEIM compared with 2.3% in the control group. Additionally, when comparing RFA with sham procedures, there were significant differences in complete eradication of both LGD (90.5% vs 22.7%, respectively) and HGD (81.0% vs 19.0%, respectively). Furthermore, disease progression in the sham group was significantly higher when compared with the RFA group (16.3% vs 3.6%, respectively). Patients with HGD, in particular, benefited from RFA in that 19.0% of those randomized to a sham procedure had progression to EAC, whereas only 2.4% of those in the ablation group had progression of disease. Patients in the RFA group underwent a mean of 3.5 treatment sessions. Adverse effects of RFA were reported in some patients, including a higher reported degree of chest discomfort compared with controls. Esophageal stricture occurred in 6.0% of ablated patients with all undergoing subsequent successful endoscopic dilation. Excellent long-term rates of eradication of dysplasia have also been reported. In a follow-up study of patients enrolled in the AIM Dysplasia Trial, 55 (98%) of the 56 patients in the RFA group with 3-year follow-up had eradication of their dysplasia.[9]

In the Surveillance versus Radiofrequency Ablation (SURF) trial, 136 patients with BE and LGD were randomized to either RFA or endoscopic surveillance.[10] The primary outcome in this study was progression to either HGD or adenocarcinoma at 3-year follow-up. Progression of disease was found to be significantly higher in patients randomized to surveillance compared with those who underwent RFA (26.5% vs 1.5%, respectively). Patients who underwent RFA had a 1.5% risk of developing of progression to EAC compared with 8.8% for patients undergoing surveillance. Additionally, 92.6% of ablated patients had complete eradication of their dysplasia compared with 27.9% in the surveillance group. Esophageal stricture occurred in 11.8% of ablated patients with successful treatment by dilation in all instances.

The AIM Dysplasia and SURF Trials provided the necessary evidence base to subsequently influence management recommendations for patients with dysplastic BE. Current clinical practice guidelines from the American College of Gastroenterology recommend the use of endoscopic therapy for patients with LGD, with endoscopic surveillance every 12 months as an acceptable alternative management strategy.[5] Furthermore, all patients with HGD are recommended to undergo endoscopic therapy unless they have a life-limiting comorbid condition. On the basis of these trials, RFA is often considered the preferred ablative therapy of choice for non-nodular dysplastic BE.

Radiofrequency Ablation for Intestinal Metaplasia and Prevention of Esophageal Adenocarcinoma

Studies evaluating endoscopic RFA in patients with BE suggest excellent long-term results.[11] In a prospective study evaluating this issue, CEIM was present in 98.4% of patients at 2.5 years and 92.0% at 5 years.[12,13] Of the patients at 5 years with intestinal metaplasia, focal RFA resulted in complete eradication.

Despite the effectiveness of RFA in most patients, some individuals may be poor initial responders to this treatment. In a study by van Vilsteren and colleagues,[14] poor initial responders, defined as less than 50% regression of intestinal metaplasia 3 months after RFA, had worse rates of eradication of metaplasia and dysplasia and required more RFA sessions over a longer period of time. Predictors of a poor response to RFA include active reflux esophagitis, scar regeneration with BE, longer antecedent history of BE, and esophageal narrowing before treatment. In another study, significant factors associated with incomplete CEIM included longer segment BE (5.5 vs 4.0 cm) and incomplete healing between treatment sessions.[15]

A large multicenter registry study published in 2015 evaluated the incidence of EAC after RFA for BE and reported that 100 (2%) of 4982 patients

developed adenocarcinoma, with 9 patients (0.2%) dying of this disease over a mean follow-up time of 2.7 years. Baseline length of BE and histology (including presence and severity of dysplasia) were significantly associated with development of EAC. The observational nature of this study and selection bias of patients healthy enough to undergo repeated sessions of RFA may help explain the particularly low incidence rates of EAC seen in this study.[16] Nevertheless, it appears that RFA significantly reduces the likelihood of patients with BE developing EAC, particularly those with HGD.

However, large studies of strictly nondysplastic BE suggest very low rates of progression to EAC compared with older reports.[17,18] In a recent meta-analysis, the annual incidence of EAC was 0.33% in patients with nondysplastic BE and was even lower in those with short-segment BE at 0.19%.[19] Consequently, current practice guidelines do not recommend routine endoscopic therapy for patients with nondysplastic BE.[5] Rather, patients diagnosed with nondysplastic BE are recommended to undergo surveillance endoscopies with 4-quadrant biopsies at 2-cm intervals every 3 to 5 years. This remains an area of inquiry for future study; identifying patients at risk for progression versus those with indolent BE is critical to identifying which patients require early intervention.

Cost-Effectiveness of Radiofrequency Ablation

Several studies have evaluated the cost-effectiveness of RFA for treatment of BE. In a decision-analysis study using Markov modeling, initial RFA was more effective and less costly when compared with endoscopic surveillance for patients with HGD.[20] In patients with LGD, a management strategy of initial upfront RFA compared with continued surveillance with RFA performed after the development of HGD led to an incremental cost-effectiveness ratio of $18,231/quality-adjusted life-year, suggesting this may be cost-effective. A follow-up analysis of data from the SURF trial also evaluated treatment costs of patients with LGD. The investigators found ablation for these patients to be more expensive than surveillance during the trial period. Subsequently, in estimates derived from bootstrap analyses, they found ablation of patients with LGD to be $40,915 per prevented event when the subsequent downstream costs of treating progression to HGD or adenocarcinoma were included.[21]

Finally, evidence suggests that RFA for patients with BE without dysplasia may not be cost-effective and too expensive to implement on a broad scale.[20] Considering the very low rates of progression of nondysplastic BE to EAC in conjunction with the prohibitive cost of endoscopic ablation for these patients, interval surveillance endoscopy for nondysplastic BE, and not RFA, continues to be recommended.[5]

Radiofrequency Ablation and Endoscopic Mucosal Resection

The use of endoscopic mucosal resection (EMR) is often used in patients with nodular disease or early EAC for which RFA alone would be ineffective. EMR may be used in patients with non-nodular dysplastic BE as well. In patients with HGD without circumferential disease, patients are oftentimes managed with a strategy of combined EMR followed by RFA with studies reporting excellent rates of eradication for both metaplastic and neoplastic disease.[22,23] Recently, several studies and meta-analyses have suggested that RFA may be equally effective to EMR for the treatment of dysplastic BE with a significantly lower overall adverse event and stricture rate.[22,24,25] In one study, the relative risk for adverse events was 4.4 for those treated with EMR compared with those with RFA alone.[25] In another "real-world"

evaluation of registry data, the use of EMR before RFA did not improve eradication rates of dysplasia or offer any additional benefit.[22] However, caution must be used in interpreting these data, as factors such as BE segment length and circumferential versus focal disease affect both the relative benefit and, conversely, complication rates after EMR. Further discussion regarding the use of EMR and its indications and outcomes in the setting of dysplastic BE and early EAC may be found elsewhere in this issue.

CRYOABLATION

Cryoablation is a relatively new technology that has gained increasing acceptance as a tool for ablation in patients with BE, with or without dysplasia, as well as those with early EAC. Use of this modality for the treatment of patients with BE was first reported in 2005.[26] Although there are variations in practice, the most commonly reported current form of this technology uses an endoscopic spray catheter to deliver medical-grade liquid nitrogen at a temperature of -196°C at low pressures (**Fig. 2**). Alternatively, cryoablation using an endoscopic balloon delivery system has also been described.[27] Endoscopists may administer multiple freeze cycles at targeted tissue

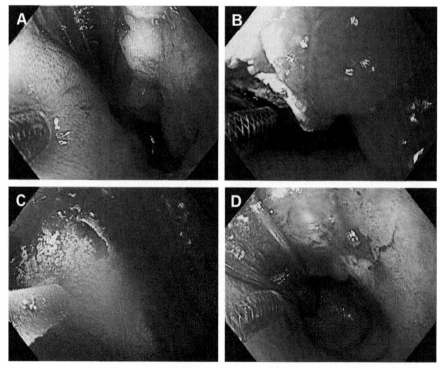

Fig. 2. Liquid nitrogen spray cryotherapy performed in a patient with BE and dysplasia. (*A*) Dysplastic segment in background of BE seen anteriorly. (*B, C*) Targeted delivery of liquid nitrogen spray cryotherapy. (*D*) Posttreatment after liquid nitrogen spray cryotherapy.

sites based on their individual protocols before moving to another anatomic location. Similar to RFA, cryoablation typically requires multiple treatment sessions several weeks to months apart before CEIM or eradication of dysplasia is achieved.

Cryoablation for Dysplastic Barrett's Esophagus

In the largest prospective study to date on spray cryotherapy, Ghorbani and colleagues[28] reported results from the National Cryospray Registry examining a total of 96 patients with dysplastic BE. Patients were treated with liquid nitrogen spray cryotherapy every 2 to 3 months until eradication was achieved with subsequent surveillance endoscopies up to 2 years afterward. In patients with LGD, complete eradication of dysplasia was achieved in 91% and CEIM occurred in 61%. In those with HGD, eradication rates of dysplasia and metaplasia occurred in 81% and 65%, respectively. Patients with short-segment BE experienced even higher rates of eradication of any dysplasia and metaplasia (97% and 77%, respectively).

In one of the largest retrospective studies published, 98 patients with BE and HGD underwent liquid nitrogen spray cryotherapy with 60 completing all planned treatment sessions. There was complete eradication of HGD in 58 (97%) patients and eradication of all dysplasia in 52 (87%) patients.[29] Gosain and colleagues[30] found that 32 (100%) of 32 patients with BE and HGD treated with liquid nitrogen spray cryotherapy had complete eradication of their dysplasia at 2-year follow-up. Recurrence of dysplasia occurred in 6 patients (18%) with complete eradication again achieved after repeat cryotherapy in 5 patients and progression to adenocarcinoma in 1 patient.

Recently, long-term outcomes of spray cryotherapy in patients with HGD and intramucosal adenocarcinoma, including those treated with EMR, were reported. At 5 years, complete eradication of HGD, dysplasia, and intestinal metaplasia were 93%, 88%, and 75%, respectively. In patients who achieved CEIM, the incidence of recurrent HGD/intramucosal adenocarcinoma was 1.4% per person-year.[31]

These studies suggest cryoablation is a reasonable alternative to RFA for the treatment of dysplastic BE. However, the uncontrolled nature of these studies, differences in patient selection between analyses, and variation in ablation techniques for both cryotherapy and RFA render any generalizations between these 2 modalities problematic.

Cryoablation for Esophageal Adenocarcinoma and as Salvage Therapy

The use of spray cryotherapy in patients with EAC has also been described.[32–34] Tsai and colleagues[34] reported results from a multicenter registry of 88 patients with T1a-T2 esophageal cancer. With a mean follow-up of 18.4 months, patient complete response rates were 76.3% for T1a, 45.8% for T1b, 66.2% for unspecified T1, and 6.7% for T2 disease. No perforations occurred and strictures were reported in 13.6% of patients, a quarter of whom had strictures before beginning treatment.

Additionally, cryotherapy has been used after EMR for intramucosal adenocarcinoma with results seemingly comparable to the more conventional approach of RFA after EMR.[35] Finally, liquid nitrogen spray cryotherapy also has been used as a salvage therapy after prior failed RFA for BE.[36]

Safety of Cryoablation

Cryoablation is generally well-tolerated. In a study of 77 patients who underwent 323 cryoablations, patient symptoms were evaluated 1 to 10 days after treatment.[37] The most common postprocedural complaints included chest pain (17.6%), dysphagia (13.3%), odynophagia (12.1%), and sore throat (9.6%), with no side effects noted in 48% of procedures. Symptoms occurred more commonly in patients with BE segments 6 cm or longer. There was one gastric perforation that occurred in a patient with a history of Marfan syndrome and 3 patients developed esophageal stricture with successful treatment by endoscopic dilation.

In the largest retrospective study to date on endoscopic spray cryotherapy, 98 patients underwent 333 treatments with no perforations occurring.[29] Adverse events included strictures developing in 3 patients, chest pain requiring narcotics in 2 patients, and development of gastrointestinal bleeding in 1 patient requiring hospitalization.

Cryoablation with Carbon Dioxide

Endoscopic cryotherapy with use of pressurized carbon dioxide (CO_2), as opposed to liquid nitrogen, has also been described. This approach appears to be efficacious for CEIM, although long-term outcomes are lacking.[38] Nevertheless, reports of the use of CO_2 cryotherapy in HGD and neoplasia in both treatment-naïve patients as well as a rescue option for previously treated individuals with persistent or recurrent disease suggests this may be an effective endoscopic approach to ablation.[39]

Further controlled studies are needed for direct comparisons of cryotherapy, both liquid nitrogen and CO_2, and RFA to determine the most appropriate treatment regimen for patients with dysplastic BE and early EAC.

POSTTREATMENT SURVEILLANCE

Although the initial success rates from endoscopic ablation of intestinal metaplasia and dysplasia are high, recurrence of disease is not uncommon.[40] In a study of patients with dysplastic BE or intramucosal adenocarcinoma who underwent RFA, the incidence of disease recurrence was 5.2% per year and progression occurred in 1.9% per year.[41] In a more recent study, the incidence rate of recurrent intestinal metaplasia or dysplasia after RFA was 9.6% per year with 58% of patients achieving CEIM after further ablation. However, 1.8% of patients did progress to invasive EAC.[42]

Patients with longer baseline segments of BE appear to be at higher risk for recurrence. Studies suggest dysplastic recurrences occur most often at the gastroesophageal junction and cardia, with most recurrences not visible on endoscopy but rather detected on random biopsies.[42,43]

Clinical practice guidelines from the American College of Gastroenterology recommend endoscopic surveillance in patients successfully treated with ablation and with CEIM.[5] For those patients with a history of HGD or intramucosal carcinoma before ablation, current recommendations are endoscopic surveillance every 3 months for the first year and every 6 months for the second year after eradication. If no evidence of disease recurrence is present, they should be surveilled annually going forward. For those with LGD, recommendations after ablation are surveillance every 6 months for the first year followed by annual endoscopies.

SUMMARY

The use of endoscopic therapies for the management of BE continues to evolve. Multicenter randomized controlled trials have demonstrated efficacy in the use of RFA to prevent progression of disease in patients with dysplastic BE. In recent years, several retrospective and prospective studies have suggested that cryoablation may be yet another valuable tool to add to the endoscopists' armamentarium for the eradication of BE. As these technologies increasingly become incorporated into use by endoscopists, we are left with many remaining questions. In particular, understanding the precise roles that RFA, cryoablation,

and EMR have in patients with nondysplastic BE at high risk of progression as well as those with dysplasia or early EAC has yet to be fully elucidated. Nevertheless, these advancements have allowed endoscopists to offer patients a minimally invasive therapy with which to treat esophageal metaplasia and dysplasia, and in some cases, prevent the occurrence of invasive EAC.

REFERENCES

1. Rubenstein JH, Morgenstern H, Appelman H, et al. Prediction of Barrett's esophagus among men. Am J Gastroenterol 2013;108(3):353–62.
2. El-Serag HB, Sweet S, Winchester CC, et al. Update on the epidemiology of gastro-oesophageal reflux disease: a systematic review. Gut 2014; 63(6):871–80.
3. Hayeck TJ, Kong CY, Spechler SJ, et al. The prevalence of Barrett's esophagus in the US: estimates from a simulation model confirmed by SEER data. Dis Esophagus 2010;23(6):451–7.
4. Garud SS, Keilin S, Cai Q, et al. Diagnosis and management of Barrett's esophagus for the endoscopist. Therap Adv Gastroenterol 2010;3(4):227–38.
5. Shaheen NJ, Falk GW, Iyer PG, et al, American College of Gastroenterology. ACG clinical guideline: diagnosis and management of Barrett's esophagus. Am J Gastroenterol 2016;111(1):30–50.
6. Sharma P, Dent J, Armstrong D, et al. The development and validation of an endoscopic grading system for Barrett's esophagus: the Prague C & M criteria. Gastroenterology 2006;131(5):1392–9.
7. Fudman DI, Lightdale CJ, Poneros JM, et al. Positive correlation between endoscopist radiofrequency ablation volume and response rates in Barrett's esophagus. Gastrointest Endosc 2014;80(1):71–7.
8. Shaheen NJ, Sharma P, Overholt BF, et al. Radiofrequency ablation in Barrett's esophagus with dysplasia. N Engl J Med 2009;360(22):2277–88.
9. Shaheen NJ, Overholt BF, Sampliner RE, et al. Durability of radiofrequency ablation in Barrett's esophagus with dysplasia. Gastroenterology 2011; 141(2):460–8.
10. Phoa KN, van Vilsteren FG, Weusten BL, et al. Radiofrequency ablation vs endoscopic surveillance for patients with Barrett esophagus and low-grade dysplasia: a randomized clinical trial. JAMA 2014; 311(12):1209–17.
11. Orman ES, Li N, Shaheen NJ. Efficacy and durability of radiofrequency ablation for Barrett's esophagus: systematic review and meta-analysis. Clin Gastroenterol Hepatol 2013;11(10):1245–55.
12. Fleischer DE, Overholt BF, Sharma VK, et al. Endoscopic ablation of Barrett's esophagus: a multicenter study with 2.5-year follow-up. Gastrointest Endosc 2008;68(5):867–76.

13. Fleischer DE, Overholt BF, Sharma VK, et al. Endoscopic radiofrequency ablation for Barrett's esophagus: 5-year outcomes from a prospective multicenter trial. Endoscopy 2010;42(10):781–9.

14. van Vilsteren FG, Alvarez Herrero L, Pouw RE, et al. Predictive factors for initial treatment response after circumferential radiofrequency ablation for Barrett's esophagus with early neoplasia: a prospective multicenter study. Endoscopy 2013;45(7):516–25.

15. Bulsiewicz WJ, Kim HP, Dellon ES, et al. Safety and efficacy of endoscopic mucosal therapy with radiofrequency ablation for patients with neoplastic Barrett's esophagus. Clin Gastroenterol Hepatol 2013; 11(6):636–42.

16. Wolf WA, Pasricha S, Cotton C, et al. Incidence of esophageal adenocarcinoma and causes of mortality after radiofrequency ablation of Barrett's esophagus. Gastroenterology 2015;149(7):1752–61.e1.

17. Hvid-Jensen F, Pedersen L, Drewes AM, et al. Incidence of adenocarcinoma among patients with Barrett's esophagus. N Engl J Med 2011;365(15): 1375–83.

18. Wani S, Falk G, Hall M, et al. Patients with nondysplastic Barrett's esophagus have low risks for developing dysplasia or esophageal adenocarcinoma. Clin Gastroenterol Hepatol 2011;9(3):220–7 [quiz: e26].

19. Desai TK, Krishnan K, Samala N, et al. The incidence of oesophageal adenocarcinoma in nondysplastic Barrett's oesophagus: a meta-analysis. Gut 2012;61(7):970–6.

20. Hur C, Choi SE, Rubenstein JH, et al. The cost effectiveness of radiofrequency ablation for Barrett's esophagus. Gastroenterology 2012;143(3):567–75.

21. Phoa KN, Rosmolen WD, Weusten B, et al. The cost-effectiveness of radiofrequency ablation for Barrett's esophagus with low-grade dysplasia: results from a randomized controlled trial (SURF trial). Gastrointest Endosc 2017;86(1):120–9.e2.

22. Haidry RJ, Dunn JM, Butt MA, et al. Radiofrequency ablation and endoscopic mucosal resection for dysplastic Barrett's esophagus and early esophageal adenocarcinoma: outcomes of the UK National Halo RFA Registry. Gastroenterology 2013;145(1): 87–95.

23. Phoa KN, Pouw RE, Bisschops R, et al. Multimodality endoscopic eradication for neoplastic Barrett oesophagus: results of an European multicentre study (EURO-II). Gut 2016;65(4):555–62.

24. Chadwick G, Groene O, Markar SR, et al. Systematic review comparing radiofrequency ablation and complete endoscopic resection in treating dysplastic Barrett's esophagus: a critical assessment of histologic outcomes and adverse events. Gastrointest Endosc 2014;79(5):718–31.e3.

25. Qumseya BJ, Wani S, Desai M, et al. Adverse events after radiofrequency ablation in patients with Barrett's esophagus: a systematic review and meta-analysis. Clin Gastroenterol Hepatol 2016; 14(8):1086–95.e6.

26. Johnston MH, Eastone JA, Horwhat JD, et al. Cryoablation of Barrett's esophagus: a pilot study. Gastrointest Endosc 2005;62(6):842–8.

27. Scholvinck DW, Kunzli HT, Kestens C, et al. Treatment of Barrett's esophagus with a novel focal cryoablation device: a safety and feasibility study. Endoscopy 2015;47(12):1106–12.

28. Ghorbani S, Tsai FC, Greenwald BD, et al. Safety and efficacy of endoscopic spray cryotherapy for Barrett's dysplasia: results of the National Cryospray Registry. Dis Esophagus 2016;29(3):241–7.

29. Shaheen NJ, Greenwald BD, Peery AF, et al. Safety and efficacy of endoscopic spray cryotherapy for Barrett's esophagus with high-grade dysplasia. Gastrointest Endosc 2010;71(4):680–5.

30. Gosain S, Mercer K, Twaddell WS, et al. Liquid nitrogen spray cryotherapy in Barrett's esophagus with high-grade dysplasia: long-term results. Gastrointest Endosc 2013;78(2):260–5.

31. Ramay FH, Cui Q, Greenwald BD. Outcomes after liquid nitrogen spray cryotherapy in Barrett's esophagus-associated high-grade dysplasia and intramucosal adenocarcinoma: 5-year follow-up. Gastrointest Endosc 2017;86(4):626–32.

32. Dumot JA, Vargo JJ 2nd, Falk GW, et al. An open-label, prospective trial of cryospray ablation for Barrett's esophagus high-grade dysplasia and early esophageal cancer in high-risk patients. Gastrointest Endosc 2009;70(4):635–44.

33. Greenwald BD, Dumot JA, Abrams JA, et al. Endoscopic spray cryotherapy for esophageal cancer: safety and efficacy. Gastrointest Endosc 2010; 71(4):686–93.

34. Tsai FC, Ghorbani S, Greenwald BD, et al. Safety and efficacy of endoscopic spray cryotherapy for esophageal cancer. Dis Esophagus 2017; 30(11):1–7.

35. Trindade AJ, Pleskow DK, Sengupta N, et al. Efficacy of liquid nitrogen cryotherapy for Barrett's esophagus after endoscopic resection of intramucosal cancer: a multicenter study. J Gastroenterol Hepatol 2018;33(2):461–5.

36. Trindade AJ, Inamdar S, Kothari S, et al. Feasibility of liquid nitrogen cryotherapy after failed radiofrequency ablation for Barrett's esophagus. Dig Endosc 2017;29(6):680–5.

37. Greenwald BD, Dumot JA, Horwhat JD, et al. Safety, tolerability, and efficacy of endoscopic low-pressure liquid nitrogen spray cryotherapy in the esophagus. Dis Esophagus 2010;23(1):13–9.

38. Xue HB, Tan HH, Liu WZ, et al. A pilot study of endoscopic spray cryotherapy by pressurized carbon dioxide gas for Barrett's esophagus. Endoscopy 2011; 43(5):379–85.

39. Canto MI, Shin EJ, Khashab MA, et al. Safety and efficacy of carbon dioxide cryotherapy for treatment of neoplastic Barrett's esophagus. Endoscopy 2015; 47(7):582–91.

40. Gupta M, Iyer PG, Lutzke L, et al. Recurrence of esophageal intestinal metaplasia after endoscopic mucosal resection and radiofrequency ablation of Barrett's esophagus: results from a US Multicenter Consortium. Gastroenterology 2013;145(1):79–86.e1.

41. Orman ES, Kim HP, Bulsiewicz WJ, et al. Intestinal metaplasia recurs infrequently in patients successfully treated for Barrett's esophagus with radiofrequency ablation. Am J Gastroenterol 2013;108(2):187–95 [quiz: 196].

42. Guthikonda A, Cotton CC, Madanick RD, et al. Clinical outcomes following recurrence of intestinal metaplasia after successful treatment of Barrett's esophagus with radiofrequency ablation. Am J Gastroenterol 2017;112(1):87–94.

43. Vaccaro BJ, Gonzalez S, Poneros JM, et al. Detection of intestinal metaplasia after successful eradication of Barrett's esophagus with radiofrequency ablation. Dig Dis Sci 2011;56(7): 1996–2000.

Endoscopic Resection in the Esophagus

Andrew F. Feczko, MD, Brian E. Louie, MD, MHA, MPH, FRCSC, FACS*

KEYWORDS

- Esophageal cancer • Endoscopic resection • Endoscopic mucosal resection
- Endoscopic submucosal dissection

KEY POINTS

- Endoscopic resection is commonly used as first-line treatment of most intramucosal esophageal cancers and high-grade dysplasia.
- Endoscopic mucosal resection and endoscopic submucosal dissection are both applicable endoscopic techniques but differ in regard to speed, opportunity for en bloc resection, and skill required.
- There are few studies that directly compare outcomes following endoscopic resection techniques for superficial esophageal cancer.
- Endoscopic resection is superior to esophagectomy for early superficial cancers in terms of complications and length of stay. Oncologic outcomes seem equivalent for early and appropriately staged disease.

INTRODUCTION

The development of esophageal adenocarcinoma is based on an inflammatory pathway that begins with normal squamous mucosa undergoing transformation to intestinal metaplasia or Barrett esophagus (BE). With increasing genetic changes and ongoing inflammation from chronic gastroesophageal reflux disease (GERD), dysplastic changes ensue and progress to cancer. This understanding has led to improved surveillance in this setting and early identification of lesions isolated to the mucosa amenable to curative resection using advanced endoscopic surgical techniques.[1–4]

Advanced endoscopic techniques have supplanted more traditional approaches to many of the benign and malignant conditions of the esophagus and stomach. BE with high-grade dysplasia (HGD) and intramucosal esophageal cancer (IMC) were among the first 2 pathologic conditions to move toward an endoscopic approach with radiofrequency ablation (RFA) and endoscopic resection (ER). These techniques are now

considered first-line treatment and standard of care in appropriately selected patients. This article reviews the techniques and variations of endoscopic mucosal resection (EMR) and endoscopic submucosal dissection (ESD). Common complications and their frequency with each technique are discussed. This involves a review of the current literature describing the relative advantages and disadvantages of each technique, and comparing the outcomes between endoscopic techniques and esophagectomy.

PRINCIPLES OF ENDOSCOPIC RESECTION

The principles underlying ER of HGD and IMC are based on experience and knowledge gained from radical resection of these tumors. The idea that esophageal cancer could be treated with anything less than esophagectomy seemed impossible because of the rich and easily accessed esophageal submucosal lymphatic plexus leading to early metastatic nodal spread. Analysis of radical esophagectomy specimens with extensive

Disclosure Statement: The authors have nothing to disclose.
Division of Thoracic Surgery, Swedish Cancer Institute, 1101 Madison Avenue, Seattle, WA 98104, USA
* Corresponding author.
E-mail address: BRIAN.LOUIE@SWEDISH.ORG

Thorac Surg Clin 28 (2018) 481–497
https://doi.org/10.1016/j.thorsurg.2018.07.006

lymphadenectomies demonstrated a progressive risk of nodal metastases based on the depth of the lesion, such that intramucosal tumors (tumors superficial to the muscularis mucosa; tumor stage [T]1a) and HGD had few, if any, lymph node metastases (0%–1.3%). Conversely, lesions involving the submucosa (T1b) had high rates of lymph node involvement (12%–34%). The likelihood of lymph node metastasis continues to increase with T2 (43%), T3 (77.2%), and T4 tumors (66.7%).[1,5–8] Understanding this relationship, it has been shown that superficial mucosal tumors can be safely resected endoscopically without further evaluating the draining lymph nodes.

Endoscopic Mucosal Resection

EMR is an endoscopic procedure that allows removal of the mucosa and submucosa of the esophagus or stomach by creating a pseudopolyp of tissue containing the diseased mucosa. The mucosa is suctioned into a cap placed on the distal end of the endoscope and the polyp is elevated by applying a rubber band. This is then resected using a snare (**Fig. 1**). EMR has both diagnostic and therapeutic functions. Complete removal of a lesion of the mucosa may result in cure; however, a lesion that demonstrates deeper invasion provides accurate tumor staging for a new cancer.

The technique has been used for the resection of nodular BE, early esophageal adenocarcinoma, and early squamous cell carcinoma (T1a).[9–12] Professional societies recommend using EMR for lesions 20 mm or smaller, involving less than one-third the circumference of the esophagus, and limited to the submucosa.[11] It has been the authors' practice to apply these guidelines particularly when a lesion is small enough for complete resection as a single specimen. Despite these recommendations, EMR is frequently used for the removal of lesions larger than 2 cm, with debate regarding the oncologic rigor of this practice. Complete resection of superficial lesions by EMR (negative deep and radial margins) is curative; however, this can only be determined following resection and pathologic review.

ENDOSCOPIC MUCOSAL RESECTION TECHNIQUES

EMR can be performed under moderate sedation or general anesthesia based on the planned duration of the procedure, need for multiple endoscope passes, or the use of larger endoscope distal caps. In addition to white light and electronic chromoendoscopy imaging capabilities and EMR instruments, it is useful to have coagulation forceps and endoclips readily available for hemostasis and control of microperforations. The procedure is

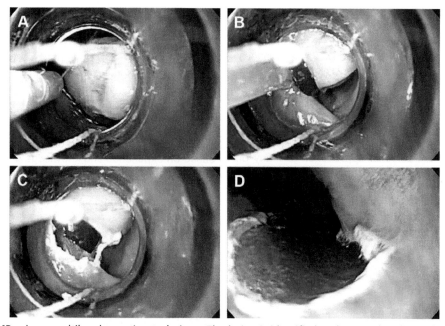

Fig. 1. EMR using a multiband resection technique. The lesion is identified and a pseudopolyp is developed by applying a band to the involved mucosa (*A*). Once the mucosa is elevated, a snare cautery is used to encircle and divide the stalk below the band (*B*) and (*C*). The technique is applied repeatedly until all the involved mucosa is resected. The ulcer bed is inspected for hemostasis (*D*).

usually completed on an outpatient basis and patients are continued on high-dose proton pump inhibitors (PPIs) until the resulting ulcer is healed.[11]

Single-Band Resection

Using standard variceal banding equipment, the lesion is suctioned and banded creating a pseudopolyp. The endoscope is then withdrawn, and the banding device removed. The endoscope is then reinserted, and the lesion is amputated using a hot or cold snare above or below the band.[11] This is similar to the initial experimental procedure proposed by Inoue and Endo,[13] in which the mucosa is pulled into a snare using a grasping forceps and removed. This allows for sampling of the mucosa and submucosa, presumably without violation of the underlying muscularis propria. Equipment for this procedure is frequently already available in endoscopy suites. Single-band resection is generally used for small (<20 mm), isolated lesions owing to the time required for multiple passes of the endoscope and the availability of more efficient equipment.

Multiband Resection Technique

Multiband resection (MBR) or multiband mucosectomy differs in the use of a specialized banding device capable of delivering 4 to 10 bands before the endoscope must be removed and uses a hexagonal snare device placed through the endoscope working port for resection and retrieval of the specimen. Like the single-band technique, MBR does not require submucosal injection (see **Fig. 1**). The use of this device improves the efficiency of EMR compared with the single-band technique and makes piecemeal resection of lesions larger than 2 cm tenable. Because the endoscope does not have to be withdrawn multiple times, it is possible to complete the resection with moderate sedation; however, general anesthesia may be used if a longer procedure is anticipated.

Large-Cap Endoscopic Mucosal Resection

Large-cap resection (LCR) differs from the aforementioned techniques in that the lesion is raised off the underlying muscle by the injection of saline (with or without epinephrine or methylene blue) or a hydrogel solution into the submucosa. A plastic cap (usually an oblique cap in esophageal EMR, in which the endoscope is parallel to the resection plane) is applied to the tip of the endoscope and a device-specific snare is positioned at the cap opening. Suction is applied to the lifted lesion and, once captured within the cap, the snare is tightened and cautery applied (**Fig. 2**). The specimen is then retrieved. LCR has been shown to achieve en bloc resection of lesions slightly larger than 2 cm.[14]

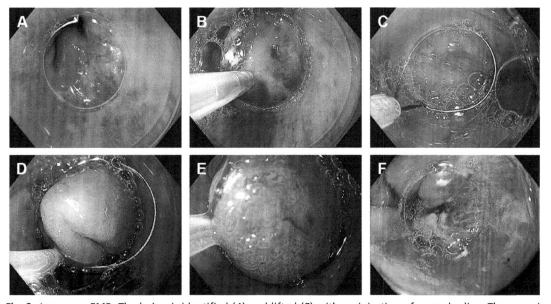

Fig. 2. Large-cap EMR. The lesion is identified (*A*) and lifted (*B*) with an injection of normal saline. The snare is positioned at the end of the cap using a specifically designed ridge to control deployment (*C*). Suction is applied and the lesion containing mucosa is pulled into the snare and cap (*D*). Cautery is applied (*E*), amputating the pseudopolyp. The endoscope is removed as a unit and the specimen submitted for pathologic assessment. The resection site is inspected for hemostasis (*F*) and to determine the need for additional resection.

Comparison of endoscopic mucosal resection techniques

Comparative data among different EMR techniques are limited. One randomized controlled trial by Pouw and colleagues[14] compared the efficiency and safety of endoscopic LCR versus the use of an MBR. The use of an MBR was significantly faster (34 vs 50 minutes, $P = .02$) and lower cost than cap resection. Safety between the 2 procedures was similar but with a not statistically significant trend toward increased perforation with cap resection (3 perforations vs 1 perforation with MBR). All complications were managed endoscopically. The argument has been made that LCR is a better oncologic choice because it captures larger pieces of mucosa compared with the banded techniques and avoids the need for piecemeal resections. Piecemeal resection may increase rates of the unrecognized resection margin class (R)1 at the lateral margins of a specimen and there are some data to suggest that piecemeal resection is a risk factor for local recurrence of cancer.[15]

Results of endoscopic mucosal resection

In the literature, rates of complete local remission for neoplasia (R0 resection of HGD or IMC) following EMR ranges from 80% to 99%.[3,15–18] Exact comparisons across studies are difficult given variation in resection plus ablation protocols and subsequent endoscopic surveillance. The adoption of different formats of mucosal ablation (photodynamic therapy [PDT], argon plasma coagulation [APC], and RFA) for destruction of residual BE occurred over the course of many of these studies, most without a consistent technology to supplement EMR.[15,16,19] The largest and longest series by Pech and colleagues[16] retrospectively followed 1000 subjects after EMR and ablation of HGD or IMC and nondysplastic BE with an initial complete remission rate of 96.3%. Over 5 years, recurrence occurred in 140 subjects with 115 successfully treated with repeat EMR, leading to a long-term remission rate of 93.8%. Of the 15% to 30% of subjects who developed recurrences on surveillance endoscopies in other studies, 82% to 85% were successfully treated with repeat EMR.[15,16,18] Disease-free survival is reported between 87% and 100%[15,16] (Table 1).

Many of the earlier and larger trials of EMR emphasized successful resection of HGD and intramucosal neoplasms without specifically commenting on existing or persistent intestinal metaplasia. The Wiesbaden group used empiric ablative therapies and continued PPI therapy after EMR to address residual BE but did not report eradication rates in their studies.[3,15,16,18] Compared with the high complete resection rates for dysplastic or neoplastic lesions (85%–100%) with EMR, rates of complete response to therapy for intestinal metaplasia range between 73% and 83% with EMR or EMR plus RFA.[20–22]

Major complications associated with EMR are rare and generally are managed endoscopically (see Table 1). Most bleeding either requires no treatment or responds readily to endoscopic injection or clipping (11%–32%). Rarely is bleeding considered a major adverse event, qualifying only with a hemoglobin decrease of greater than 2 g/dL or a transfusion requirement (1.4% of subjects in 1 series).[10,11,16] Perforations are similarly uncommon (0%–2% of cases), and are either directly identified or are diagnosed based on the development of subcutaneous emphysema, pneumomediastinum, or pneumothorax. Endoscopic intervention is usually sufficient (endoclips or esophageal stenting) with antibiotics and a period of nothing by mouth. Rarely, perforations lead to mediastinitis requiring surgical drainage.[17] Development of a stricture depends on the extent of mucosal resection, with the frequency approaching 100% as the resection becomes circumferential and the number of lesions resected increases. Strictures typically respond to endoscopic therapy, although repeat dilations may be necessary.[15,16,19,21]

ENDOSCOPIC SUBMUCOSAL DISSECTION
Indications

ESD was initially developed in Japan for the management of early-stage gastric tumors and is now applied throughout the gastrointestinal tract for the local resection of esophageal, gastric, and colorectal malignancies. ESD allows for en bloc resection of larger lesions (>1.5–2 cm) or lesions contained within larger areas of metaplastic or dysplastic esophageal mucosa, avoiding the need for piecemeal resections. In Japan, ESD is generally favored as first-line endoscopic therapy for resection of esophageal intramucosal lesions. The Japanese Society of Gastroenterology guidelines recommend ESD for lesions involving less than two-thirds of the esophageal lumen and recommend ESD as a relative indication when lesions involve less than 200 μm of submucosa.[23] ESD is also recommended as treatment following failed EMR and for lesions with poor lifting (lesions do not easily form a pseudopolyp with banding) requiring submucosal injection.[10] Broad enthusiasm for ESD is tempered by a greater technical challenge (fine dissection in a relatively small lumen and difficulty accessing the appropriate submucosal plane) and a correspondingly longer procedure time when compared with EMR.

Table 1
Major studies describing the effectiveness and outcomes of endoscopic mucosal resection

First Author, Year	Number of Subjects Undergoing EMR	Complete Local Remission Rate	Endoscopic Failure Rate	Long-Term Cure Rate	Ablative Therapy	Average Number of Procedures Required per Subject	Median Follow-up Period	Recurrence Rate	Mortality	Complications and Treatment
May et al,[18] 2002	115	108/110 subjects (98%)	2/110 (1.8%)	107/110 (97.2%)	PDT, APC	2	34 mo	34/110 (30%) 33 (97%), successful repeat endoscopic treatment	97/110 (88%) OS 1089/110 (99%) DFS	5 bleeding episodes, n = 5, no treatment 3 stenoses, n = 3, endoscopic treatment 0 perforations
Pech et al,[15] 2008	349	337/349 (96.6%)	13/337 (3.7%)	330/349 (94.5%)	ER, ER + PDT, PDT, APC	2.1	63.0 mo	74/344 (21.5%) 63/74 (85%), successful repeat endoscopic treatment	84% OS 5-y survival rate 100% DFS 5-y survival	Significant bleeding (Hg decrease >2 g/dL), n = 2 Minor bleeding, n = 40 Stenosis, n = 15 odynophagia, n = 1
Ell et al,[3] 2007	100	99/100 (99%)	1/100 (1%)	99/100 (99%)	APC, PDT	1.5	37 mo	11/144 (7%) All subjects successfully treated endoscopically	98/100 (98%) OS 100% DFS	Minor bleeding, n = 11
Pech et al,[16] 2014	1000	963/1000 (96.3%)	42/1000 (4.2%)	938/1000 (93.8%)	APC, PDT	1	56 mo	140/1000 (14.5%) 115/140 (82.1%), successful repeat endoscopic treatment	91.5% 5-y OS 2/1000 (0.2%) tumor-related deaths 87.1% 5-y DFS	15/1000 (1.5%) major complications (bleeding n = 14, perforation n = 1) 13/1000 (1.3%) Minor complications (stenosis req dilation, n = 13)

(continued on next page)

Table 1
(continued)

First Author, Year	Number of Subjects Undergoing EMR	Complete Local Remission Rate	Endoscopic Failure Rate	Long-Term Cure Rate	Ablative Therapy	Average Number of Procedures Required per Subject	Median Follow-up Period	Recurrence Rate	Mortality	Complications and Treatment
Oliphant et al,[19] 2014	72	59/72 (82%)	Not reported	64/72 (88.9%)	APC, PDT, RFA	4	38 mo	8/63 (12.7%), subjects with HGD progressed to submucosal cancer	Not reported	Perforation, n = 1 (endoscopic management) Stricture, n = 6 (endoscopic dilation)
Konda et al,[17] 2014	107	86/107 (80%)	21/107 (20%)	66/74 (89.2%)	RFA	Not reported	33 mo	8/74 (10.8%)	1 procedure-related mortality	Perforations, 2/107 (see notes) Strictures requiring dilation, 40/107 (37.8%)

Complete local remission rate refers to successful resection of dysplastic or neoplastic lesions at follow-up endoscopy. Endoscopic failure rate refers to cases were ER was attempted but esophagectomy was ultimately required for persistent disease, more advanced recurrence or significant endoscopic complication.
Abbreviations: DFS, disease-free survival; Hg, hemoglobin; Req, required; OS, overall survival.

Endoscopic Submucosal Dissection Technique

ESD is typically performed with general endotracheal anesthesia because the procedures can be technically challenging and time intensive. Once the lesion is identified with white light or chromoendoscopy imaging, a circumferential margin is marked using cautery or APC. A 5 to 10 mm margin of grossly normal epithelium is recommended for esophageal adenocarcinoma due to concern for potential subepithelial spread. Squamous cell carcinomas require a less extensive resection and marked margins are recommended between 3 and 5 mm.[10,23] Once the lesion is defined, a lifting solution is injected into the submucosal layer to better define the plane between submucosa and the underlying muscle. Some practitioners recommend performing this step after making a partial circumferential mucosal incision, exposing the submucosa, and injecting directly into this plane. Using technique-specific instruments, such as the Hybrid-Knife (Erbe USA Inc. Marietta, GA, USA), additional lifting solution can be administered to maintain the dissection plane between submucosa and muscle without having to use a dual-channel endoscope or frequently switch instruments. Multiple different dissecting, injecting, and electrocautery instruments have been developed and applied to ESD (a formal review is beyond the scope of this discussion). A transparent cap at the distal tip of the endoscope (straight, oblique, or tapered) facilitates dissection by generating countertraction to lift the specimen off the muscular layer and clearly define the dissection plane. A cap also helps to maintain visualization of the target tissues while allowing the endoscope to act as a dissecting instrument. With the distal cap and endoscopic knife, the mucosa containing the target lesion is undermined. Vessels crossing in the submucosal plane are precoagulated using electrocautery or coagulation forceps because bleeding or clipping within the submucosal space can make the remainder of the dissection difficult. Once the submucosal dissection is completed, the remaining mucosal incision is completed to free the specimen. The dissection bed is inspected for hemostasis and evidence of perforation, both of which can typically be addressed endoscopically (**Fig. 3**).[10,11] Following the procedure, patients are kept on high-dose PPIs to allow the resulting ulcer to heal. If a perforation is identified or suspected, patients are admitted

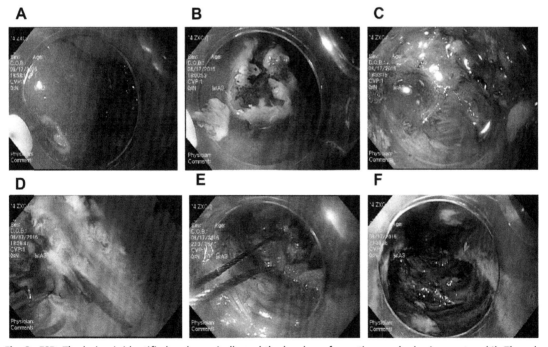

Fig. 3. ESD: The lesion is identified endoscopically and the borders of resection marked using cautery (*A*). The submucosal plane is then infiltrated with saline mixed with methylene blue to lift the lesion from the underlying muscular layer (*B*). The mucosectomy is extended to allow the endoscopic cap to be wedged in the space, developing tension to separate the submucosal fibers and muscular esophageal wall. These fibers are divided with cautery (*C*). Submucosal vessels are precoagulated with a coagulating forceps when encountered (*D*). The lesion is undermined and mucosa divided following the premarked margins. Once fully separated, the specimen is captured with a snare and removed (*E*). The remaining ulcer is inspected for residual disease and hemostasis (*F*).

and kept at nothing by mouth until a swallow study can be completed. In some centers, ESD is completed as an outpatient procedure.

A more recent advance in ESD is the application of a tunneling technique (endoscopic tunneled submucosal dissection). In this procedure, appropriate 5 mm margins around the lesion are defined with cautery or APC, and the submucosa is raised using injected saline or other solution. Once the lift is acceptable, transverse incisions are made on the proximal and distal ends of the resection margins and a submucosal tunnel is dissected from proximal to distal using the technique previously described. Once the tunnel is completed, the lateral mucosal bridges are divided until the specimen is free.[24,25] As with standard ESD, once the specimen is removed, the resulting ulcer is checked for hemostasis, exposed vessels, or perforations, and addressed endoscopically. Interest in the tunneled technique is growing with reports suggesting that modifications shorten the procedure time, bringing it on par with EMR.

RESULTS OF ENDOSCOPIC SUBMUCOSAL DISSECTION

Initial publications from Japan and Korea using ESD focused on resection of squamous cell cancers. As the technique has been explored in Western countries, experience with BE-related dysplasia and IMC has expanded.[26,27] Single-piece mucosal specimens obtained through ESD are typically larger than those obtained by EMR but vary significantly based on the lesion and experience of the operator (2–125 mm). The technical challenges associated with this procedure are reflected by longer reported procedure times (median times 45–121 minutes). Rates of en bloc resection for HGD and IMC, removal of the lesion and mucosal margin as a single specimen, are universally high with ESD (91%–100%).[28–30] R0 resection (tumor negative lateral and vertical margins), are reportedly achieved in 59% to 97% of cases. With the emphasis on lateral margins in ESD, most R1 margins occurred at the deep margin secondary to submucosal invasion. Curative resection (en bloc resection of the target lesion without poor differentiation, lymphovascular invasion [LVI], or submucosal involvement) is seen in 53% to 99% of cases (**Table 2**). Noncurative resections are referred to esophagectomy, definitive chemoradiation therapy, or no further therapy depending on the patient's comorbidities and goals.[26,28–34] Reported recurrence rates following curative ESD are generally low. In the largest series of recurrences from Park and colleagues,[32] 26 recurrences occurred following 201 curative resections (12.9%) over a 10-year experience. These recurrences were detected on surveillance endoscopy within the first 2 years following the index procedure with most managed endoscopically (APC, EMR, or repeat ESD). One subject of the 201 curative resections was referred to surgery following recurrence. Reported outcomes for tunneled ESD have been limited to small studies, with the largest being a report of 38 resections from Huang and colleagues.[35] With the tunneled technique, en bloc, complete, and curative resection rates remained high (100%, 100%, 94.7%, respectively) with no significant complications reported. The median reported procedure time was 38 minutes for tunneled ESD, which is significantly better than the median procedure time from the conventional ESD arm of the study (45 minutes, $P = .016$).

Complications associated with ESD are bleeding, perforation, and stricture (see **Table 2**). Bleeding occurs in 1.5% to 5.6% of cases, with all reported cases managed endoscopically. Only 1 group noted the need for a transfusion following a delayed bleed in 1 of 36 subjects.[29] The rate of perforation with ESD ranged from 0% to 7% of cases, with most managed during the index procedure with immediate closure of the muscular layer using endoscopic clips. Occasionally, perforation was identified after subjects developed subcutaneous emphysema or on postprocedure chest radiographs demonstrating pneumomediastinum. Of the studies reviewed, only 1 reported a subject requiring treatment of mediastinitis with chest drainage, antibiotics, and hospitalization.[36] Esophageal stricture following ESD is the most common complication reported, seen in 6.5% to 19% of subjects. Most strictures are successfully treated with serial balloon dilation and, in refractory cases, self-expanding stent placement. The formation of strictures correlates with the degree of circumferential resection, with greater than 50% of symptomatic strictures developing after resections involving three-fourths or more of the circumference of the esophageal mucosa.[32,37] The use of oral or locally administered steroids has been suggested to decrease the rate of post-ESD stricturing and, in 1 series, empirical use of a steroid taper protocol for resections greater than three-fourths circumference resulted in stricture in only 1 of 7 subjects who underwent 75% to 100% circumferential resections.[10,26]

Comparison of Endoscopic Resection Techniques: Endoscopic Mucosal Resection Versus Endoscopic Submucosal Dissection

EMR and ESD are recognized as viable alternatives to esophagectomy for HGD and IMC, however, it

Table 2
Major studies describing the effectiveness and outcomes of endoscopic submucosal dissection

Ablative Therapy	Average Procedure Time	Median Follow-up Period	Recurrence Rate	Mortality	Complications
APC, EMR	Mean procedure time 45 min	36 mo	26/201 (curative resection) (12.9%)	5-y OS 89.7% DFS 100% in the curative resection group	Bleeding, n = 4 (1.5%), endoscopic treatment perforation, n = 12 (4.6%), endoscopic treatment Stricture, n = 17 (6.5%), endoscopic treatment
APC	Mean procedure time 51 min	23 mo	2/27 (7%)	OS 25/27 (92.6%)	Bleeding, n = 0 Perforation, n = 2, endoscopic treatment Stricture, n = 1, endoscopic treatment
RFA	Median procedure time 88 min	10 mo	0/25	None reported	Bleeding, n = 1, endoscopic treatment Stricture, n = 7, endoscopic treatment
	Mean procedure time 80 min	22 mo	7/121 (5.8%)	DFS 98%	Bleeding, n = 2, endoscopic treatment, 1 transfusion Stricture, n = 3/143, endoscopic treatment
RFA, focal EMR	Median procedure time 121 min	11.3 mo	0/32	Not reported	Bleeding, n = 3, endoscopic treatment Stricture, n = 7, endoscopic treatment Perforation n = 1, endoscopic treatment
Not reported	tESD 38 min vs cESD 48 min	Not reported	Not reported	Not reported	Bleeding (tESD vs cESD) 0 vs 1 (1.3%) Perforation (tESD vs cESD) 0 vs 4 (5.2%) Muscular injury (tESD vs cESD) 11 (29%) vs 35 (45%)

En bloc, complete and curative resection rates are as defined in the preceding section. Endoscopic failure rate refers to subjects who underwent esophagectomy after ESD for more advanced disease or failure to obtain complete eradication with subsequent endoscopic procedures.
Abbreviations: cESD, conventional ESD; tESD, tunneled ESD.

remains unclear which technique provides the best oncologic results, with the fewest adverse events and the greatest efficiency. EMR is reported as having excellent initial (97%) and long-term complete resection rates (94%) when residual BE is ablated and recurrences are managed endoscopically.[15] A major critique of EMR, however, is that for lesions greater than 20 mm, piecemeal resection limits accurate histologic assessment of lateral margins, theoretically increasing the risk for R1 resection and recurrent disease. ESD specifically addresses this concern with en bloc resections of the target lesion, obtaining an adequate margin, and allowing accurate histologic assessment of the lateral and deep margins. Early studies comparing ESD and EMR for the resection of early squamous cancer

showed significantly higher en bloc resection and complete resection rates with ESD compared with EMR (100% vs 53%, 97% vs 78%, respectively) (**Table 3**). Curative resection rates with ESD in these studies are also significantly better than EMR (99% vs 78.3%).[30] Later comparative studies, however, are less definitive. Jin and colleagues[33] showed that, for lesions greater than 15 mm, ESD compared with EMR had a significantly higher en bloc (100% vs 44.8%, respectively) and curative resection rate (92.3% vs 41%, respectively). Howemver, for lesions less than 15 mm, curative resection rates were not statistically different (100% vs 84%, $P = .406$) and overall recurrence for all lesions was not statistically different at 3 years.[33] A 2017 randomized controlled trial of

Table 3
Direct comparison studies between endoscopic mucosal resection and endoscopic submucosal dissection

Ablative Therapy	Average Procedure Time	Median Follow-up Period	Recurrence Rate	Mortality	Complications
APC	EMR 44 min ESD 74 min	EMR 83 mo ESD 36 mo	EMR: 18/184 (9.8%) ESD: 1/116 (1%)	Disease-specific EMR: 4/184 (2%) ESD 1/116 (1%)	Perforation: 1.6% EMR vs 2.6% ESD Stenosis: 9.2% EMR vs 17.2% ESD ($P = .07$)
Not reported	Weighted mean difference of 44 min between EMR and ESD	Not reported	EMR 11.5% ESD 0.3%	Not reported	Perforation: OR ESD vs EMR 2.19 ($P = .59$) Stricture: OR ESD vs EMR 1.14 ($P = .59$) Bleeding: OR ESD vs EMR 0.74 ($P = .65$)
APC	EMR 38 min ESD 84 min	Not reported	EMR 13% at 3 y ESD 4.2% at 3 y	Not reported	Perforation: ESD 2/24 (8.3%), EMR 0 Major bleeding: ESD 4/24 (16%), EMR 1/54 (2%) Stenosis: ESD 4/24 (16%), EMR 8/54 (14.8%)
RFA	EMR 22 min ESD 54 min	3 mo	ESD 1/20 (5%)	None	Perforation: ESD 2/20, (10%), EMR 0

Abbreviation: OR, odds ratio.

ESD and EMR for HGD or IMC in BE confirmed again that ESD is superior at achieving en bloc resection; however, at 3 months follow-up, complete remission from neoplasia was the same between both groups (94% for both ESD and EMR).[36]

Understanding these data in the context of studies focused only on ESD or EMR further complicates the comparison. Data from large EMR trials tend to demonstrate excellent initial rates of complete resection, even when piecemeal resection is identified as a risk factor for recurrence.[15,16] These studies use additional endoscopic therapy, ablation of residual dysplastic mucosa (APC, RFA, PDT), and repeat EMR for recurrent lesions, and long-term remission reflects that ongoing treatment. Studies from Western institutions using ESD for the resection of BE and related neoplasia demonstrate excellent en bloc resection rates (91%–100%) but lower overall cure rates (66%–70%) when compared with older ESD trials and EMR.[28,29,37] Those studies that directly compare EMR and ESD do not clearly define how or if repeat EMR or ablative techniques were used in either arm of the trial and, therefore, accurate comparisons to how EMR is used in practice are lacking.[30,38] To further complicate comparison between these techniques, endoscopic failure rates for ESD seem to be significantly worse when EMR-only and ESD-only studies are compared (see **Tables 1** and **2**). Endoscopic failure refers to

the transition to esophagectomy after initial ER. It has been suggested that this reflects greater consistency of submucosal sampling in ESD and more patients being diagnosed with submucosal invasion greater than 200 μm and/or LVI.

The other major areas of comparison between these techniques focus on the differences in performing the procedure itself. Compared with EMR, ESD procedures are longer in both ESD-specific studies and in comparative studies against EMR. Studies from centers in East Asia generally report median time for ESD as less than 60 minutes, whereas Western centers report median procedure times greater than 60 minutes[29,31,32,37] (see **Tables 2** and **3**). As noted previously, tunneled ESD may decrease the procedure time for submucosal dissection, bringing it closer to the efficiency of EMR. Direct comparisons between EMR and tunneled ESD are lacking.

Because it is more technically challenging and involves a deeper dissection, ESD is thought to have a higher complication profile than EMR. The overall rate of complications, however, remains low (single events in some small series). Using the frequencies of adverse events across multiple studies, a rough comparison suggests that bleeding rates are similar for EMR and ESD (2.9% vs 3%) but that rates of stricture and perforation both favor EMR (ESD 10.6% vs EMR 5%, ESD 6.1% vs EMR 1%) (see **Table 3**). In both procedures, most complications are managed endoscopically with endoscopic clipping for perforations or hemostasis and epinephrine injection when appropriate. Postprocedure strictures are managed with serial dilations and stent placement in refractory cases. Frequency of stenosis is correlated with resections involving greater than 75% of the esophageal lumen for both EMR and ESD. Because ESD is specifically used for the resection of larger lesions with adequate mucosal margins as a single specimen, this rate is necessarily higher. To address this common complication and decrease the need for repeated dilations, many groups are now applying local or systemic glucocorticoids following ESD to decrease the development of symptomatic stricture.[10,25,26]

There are cases were ESD is specifically preferred when compared with EMR. In the presence of prior scar tissue, prior EMR, or ablation or with lesions suspected of invading the submucosa, the inability to lift the lesion with banding or mucosal injection may necessitate submucosal dissection.[9,10] ESD may also be a more efficient for the management of multicentric disease or lesions in long-segment BE in which the larger specimen removes microscopic multicentric dysplasia or neoplasia.

ENDOSCOPIC RESECTION AND ESOPHAGECTOMY

Classically, esophagectomy is the gold standard for resection of HGD and IMC; however, it carries a risk for significant morbidity and mortality.[39,40] ER provides local control for dysplasia and early cancers without the stresses of a major operation and hospitalization, presumably with equivalent oncologic outcomes and significant improvements in adverse events, length of stay, and cost. Esophagectomy has only been directly compared with EMR. There are currently no published reports comparing esophagectomy with ESD.

Studies comparing subjects appropriate for either esophagectomy or EMR show a 100% R0 resection rate with either transhiatal or transthoracic esophagectomy for HGD and IMC. EMR in these studies achieved complete remission in 92% to 98.7% of subjects[39–42] (**Table 4**). Multiple endoscopic procedures were required for complete resection and ablative technologies (PDT, APC, RFA) were used to clear associated dysplasia or BE (rates of residual intestinal metaplasia were not reported in these studies). Subsequent surveillance after EMR in these studies demonstrated persistent low-grade dysplasia (LGD) and HGD (LGD 15%, HGD 18%–33%), results consistent with other EMR series.[39,41] Recurrent carcinoma was seen in 6% to 12% of ERs, with most successfully managed with repeat

endoscopic procedures. When eradication rates between EMR and esophagectomy were compared after repeat resections or ablations, no statistical differences were observed.[39–42]

Rates of complication are lower with EMR than esophagectomy (EMR 13%–36%, esophagectomy 32%–41%) (see **Table 4**). Which complications are specifically reported varied across comparative studies and without consensus on which complications are considered major versus minor. All EMR complications underwent endoscopic intervention, whereas some of the complications in the esophagectomy groups (anastomotic leak, feeding jejunostomy leaks) required a return to the operating room. There were 3 cancer-related deaths reported in the comparative studies reviewed, 2 in the esophagectomy group and 1 in the EMR group.[39,40] Not surprisingly, length of stay for esophagectomy (median length of stay 8–19 days) is much longer compared with EMR, with most patients undergoing outpatient procedures or 23-hour admissions. Follow-up in the surgical cohorts ranged between 43 and 74 months. Follow-up in the EMR groups ranged from 20 months to 4 years and included varying surveillance schedules after the initial EMR. The average number of follow-up EMRs that occurred over those time periods was 2 to 7.[39,42] Cost data from 2008 showed that, including follow-up procedures, the average price of EMR ($40,000) is less than the procedure cost, hospitalization, and follow-up for esophagectomy ($66,000).[41] The success of EMR for early-stage esophageal squamous cell and adenocarcinoma (HGD; T1a), and the lower adverse effects profile, outweigh the limited benefits of radical resection with esophagectomy. Esophagectomy for more advanced disease remains an option following initial EMR if more advanced disease (T1b–T2) or advanced recurrent disease is detected.

The advantages of EMR seem to make it an obvious choice for esophageal HGD or IMC; however, there are still reasons to choose an esophagectomy for early-stage disease. For some patients, a preexisting pathologic condition may make EMR technically challenging or address malignancy while leaving a patient with poor esophageal function. A large hiatal hernia or nonfunctioning esophagus (end-stage achalasia, caustic ingestion) may be better served with an esophagectomy (vagal-sparing, transhiatal) to provide an improved functional outcome and address malignancy with 1 procedure.[43,44] When compared with esophagectomy, the low complication rate and short length of stay associated with the EMR also obscures the need for rigorous follow-up. In 1 series, 2 to 6 surveillance endoscopies were performed in the first year following EMR, not

Table 4
Studies comparing endoscopic resection and esophagectomy for dysplasia and early-stage cancer

Ablative Therapy	Median Number of Treatment Sessions for EMR	Median Follow-up Period	Recurrence Rate	Mortality	Complications
PDT, APC	No data	EMR: 20 mo Esophagectomy: 48 mo	EMR 4/62 (6%) Esophagectomy 0/32	EMR 89%, esophagectomy 93% (adjusted 4-y rate) Procedure-related mortality: EMR 1/62 (1%), esophagectomy 0/32	Major complications: 8% EMR vs 13% esophagectomy Minor complications: 31% EMR vs 63% esophagectomy
PDT	1	EMR: 43 mo Esophagectomy: 64 mo	EMR 16/114 (14%) Esophagectomy 1/46 (2%)	OS: ER 83% vs surgery 95% Cancer free survival: EMR 80% vs surgery 97%	Overall complication rate: EMR 13% vs 34% surgery
APC	2	EMR: 4.1 y Esophagectomy: 3.7 y	EMR 5/76 (6.6%) Esophagectomy: no recurrence	OS at 5 y: EMR 89% vs surgery 93% DFS at 5 y: EMR 91% vs surgery 100%	EMR: 17% had minor complications (bleeding) Surgery: 32% had major complications (anastomotic leak, PNA, cardiac problems)
APC, PDT, RFA	7	EMR: 42.6 mo Esophagectomy: 70 mo	EMR 4/36 (11%) Esophagectomy: 1/49 (2%)	Overal survival: EMR 78% vs surgery 80%	EMR: Stricture 36%, bleeding 25%, perforation 3% Surgery: 51% (41% minor, 10% major)

including additional resection or ablation procedures. This level of follow-up may not be tenable for some patients due to distance from centers with the appropriate skills or poor follow-up for other social reasons.[43] For some patients, the burden of ongoing aggressive surveillance and the concern that the cancer has not been completely removed may be a significant quality-of-life issue, outweighing the morbidity or mortality risks with open or minimally invasive esophagectomy.[43,45] As with all complex therapies, the appropriateness of a given technique should be weighed against unique patient factors and the goal to achieve the best overall outcome.

POSTRESECTION MANAGEMENT
Malignancy Management

Once mucosal lesions are resected, and residual dysplastic or metaplastic areas are ablated, the frequency of appropriate follow-up is still somewhat unclear. For confirmed intramucosal lesions (HGD; T1a) status post-EMR or post-ESD (collectively, endoscopic resection – ER), the National Comprehensive Cancer Network recommends upper endoscopy every 3 months for the first year, every 6 months for the second year, and annually thereafter indefinitely. Recurrences have been detected more than 5 years after ER and ablation and at 16 years following ablation alone.[16] Currently, there is no strong evidence to identify patients predisposed to late recurrence after ER; therefore, the authors recommend ongoing surveillance with the potential need for repeat ablation or resection in persistent or recurrent disease. For completely resected adenocarcinoma in situ (Tis) or T1a lesions, no imaging follow-up is recommended.[4] Completely resected superficial T1b lesions (<200 μm of invasion) without high-risk features can be surveilled following successful ablation (see later discussion). Annual surveillance with computed tomography chest and abdomen scan is recommended for 3 years in these patients, and the application of endoscopic ultrasound may be considered as part of endoscopic follow-up.[4] These recommendations are generally reflected in the follow-up patterns of the aforementioned studies. Data supporting these recommendations, however, are limited. There are no prospective studies showing a benefit in survival, decreased recurrence, or decreased progression to invasive cancer with the current surveillance recommendations. As the use of ER techniques becomes more prevalent, determining the effectiveness of this surveillance strategy will be important to avoid the inconvenience, risk, and cost of unnecessary procedures.

Reflux Management

Patients undergoing ER and ablation techniques for BE and mucosal esophageal adenocarcinoma are placed on high-dose acid-suppression regimens (twice daily PPIs) to allow healing of the neosquamous mucosa and to prevent recurrence of metaplastic or dysplastic epithelium secondary acid exposure. The effectiveness of this suppression strategy is questionable, with rates of intestinal metaplasia recurrence as high as 43% and some studies reporting progression to malignancy after ablation.[22,46] The application of antireflux procedures to prevent recurrence of dysplastic mucosa is an alternative to medical therapy (see later discussion).

Role for Radiofrequency Ablation or Ablative Therapies

Ablative technologies (RFA, cryotherapy, APC, and PDT) have been used in the management of dysplastic esophageal lesions alone or with other endoscopic technologies for decades. For BE and esophageal adenocarcinoma specifically, management of residual dysplasia and intestinal metaplasia is important for preventing progression to more advanced disease. (See Ravi Rajaram and Wayne L. Hofstetter's article, "Mucosal Ablation Techniques for Barrett's Esophagus and Early Esophageal Cancer," in this issue.)

Current controversies
T1b cancers ER is generally well-accepted for the management of esophageal HGD and T1a cancers. Because cancers superficial to the muscularis mucosae do not interact with the submucosal lymphatics, the rate of associated lymph node metastasis is extremely low (0%–1.3%).[8] The distinct advantage of esophagectomy in patients with deeper cancers (T1b–T2) is that

esophagectomy provides control of the primary tumor, assessment of the regional nodal beds, and potential control of early lymphatic metastases.

When all T1b esophageal tumors are considered, the rate of lymph node involvement at primary esophagectomy or as subsequent therapy following ER is significantly higher (12%–34%).[5–8] T2 tumors are even more likely to have associated lymph node metastasis, with 48.5% of patients having nodal disease in 1 series.[1] Despite concerns about the appropriateness of endoscopic therapy for more advanced tumor stage, investigators have attempted to define the tumor-specific risk factors associated with lymph node involvement and to identify which submucosal tumors may be appropriate for endoscopic management. Submucosal involvement, LVI, and poor histologic grade (grade 3) are the most commonly cited factors associated with positive lymph nodes at esophagectomy in multiple studies of T1b or T2 cancers.[5,8,47,48] Some investigators have also suggested larger lesions (>1–2 cm) may be associated with increased risk lymph node metastases[5,8,47]; however, this may reflect that larger submucosal tumors are also more likely to be associated with LVI and deeper invasion. There is some consensus, although not supported by significant data, that squamous cell tumors involving less than 200 μm or adenocarcinoma involving less than 500 μm of the submucosa with low-risk features may be amenable to ER.[4,9] As expected, with increasing numbers of risk factors for disease spread, the rate of lymph node metastasis increases.[48] To further complicate management of T1b lesions, there are some data to suggest that pathologic evaluation of these specimens may frequently overreport T1a disease as T1b disease, which occurred in 59% of cases in 1 series.[49] Additional study is certainly required in this area and, at this time, ER of T1b lesions should be approached after discussion with a multidisciplinary tumor board, including surgery, medical and radiation oncology, and gastroenterology.

Reflux control after endoscopic resection Minimally invasive antireflux surgery has a well-established role in the management of symptomatic GERD but its role in reducing progression to esophageal malignancy is less clear.[50] The increased expression of proinflammatory mediators (interleukin-8, cyclooxygenase-2) associated with reflux and the subsequent development of adenocarcinoma seems to be mitigated by effective antireflux surgery. It has been hypothesized that surgical intervention may provide more durable results after endoscopic ablation or resection, repairing the anatomic barrier to reflux, and blocking the stimulus for inflammation and metaplasia.[51,52] The small number of studies that have been carried out have shown some promise. O'Connell and Velanovich[53] reported that, in subjects who underwent endoscopic ablation with RFA followed by a Nissen fundoplication, regression of Barrett metaplasia was persistent at 1 year in 18 out of 19 (95%) of those who had an antireflux procedure compared with 21 out of 28 (75%) subjects who only underwent RFA and were continued on PPIs. A subsequent study describing the results of RFA and EMR followed by Nissen fundoplication showed that 74% of all initial histologies demonstrated complete remission of cancer, dysplasia, and intestinal metaplasia. There was no progression beyond the baseline histology and there were no recurrent cancers, although persistent BE occurred in 22% and LGD in 4%.[54] Results in this second study were similar to earlier investigations describing recurrence rates after complete ablation of intestinal metaplasia with RFA and maximum dose PPI (33% at 24 months, 43% at 33 months, and 28% at 26 months, in 3 different trials).[22,46,55] Notably, following antireflux surgery in this second study, progression of recurrent disease from metaplasia to dysplasia to cancer was lower compared with series using PPIs alone. Specifically, no instances of HGD or IMC occurred during 26 months of follow-up, an improvement compared with historical studies in which progression to HGD occurred in 8% to 11% and intramucosal or invasive cancers were found in 3% to 8% of subjects.[22,46,54]

More recent studies that have combined endoscopic therapy for BE with fundoplication support some role for antireflux surgery in the management of esophageal metaplasia, dysplasia, and early cancer. Skrobić and colleagues[56] compared recurrence of intestinal metaplasia and dysplasia following endoscopic eradication (RFA only) with either twice daily PPI (25 subjects) or Nissen fundoplication (22 subjects). Over 24 months, recurrence was seen in 20% of subjects on PPIs (1 subject LGD, 4 intestinal metaplasia) compared with 9.1% subjects who underwent fundoplication (2 subjects intestinal metaplasia) ($P = .423$). A statistically significant difference in recurrence was noted between the 2 treatment paradigms in subjects with BE segments 4 cm or greater (5 subjects in PPI group vs 2 subjects in fundoplication group, $P = .021$). Komanduri and colleagues[57] included Nissen fundoplication as part of a comprehensive endoscopic eradication algorithm for BE that included EMR and RFA followed by high-dose PPI therapy. Subjects who failed to achieve complete eradication of intestinal metaplasia after 3 RFA sessions were referred to a testing algorithm to demonstrate acidic or alkaline reflux, rule out more advanced disease, and confirm adequate motility before being offered a Nissen fundoplication. Of 48 out of 221 subjects who failed initial endoscopic therapy, 39 ultimately proceeded to antireflux surgery, with 37 (95%) achieving remission. The only significant predictor of recurrent metaplasia in their series (including those who underwent only EMR plus PPI or proceeded to surgery) was the presence of a hiatal hernia.

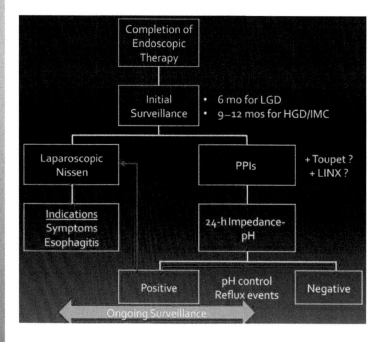

Fig. 4. Suggested algorithm for the management of persistent esophageal dysplasia following initial ER and ablation. Patients are continued on PPIs following endoscopic therapy. Those with recurrent or persistent disease at follow-up are referred for 24-hour impedance testing to evaluate for ongoing reflux. Those with evidence of clinically relevant reflux are then referred to laparoscopic Nissen fundoplication. Patients with symptomatic esophagitis before ER and recurrent or persistent disease are directly referred to fundoplication. The role of magnetic lower esophageal sphincter augmentation (LINX) or a partial 270° (Toupet) wrap for asymptomatic or mildly symptomatic individuals with persistent dysplasia is unknown but may represent an alternative to medical management of ongoing symptomatic reflux.

It is the authors' practice to make our decision to perform antireflux surgery after a period of post-EMR or ablation surveillance. Patients with persistent GERD symptoms or esophagitis despite maximal dose PPIs are offered antireflux surgery. Whereas, patients without symptoms on maximal PPI therapy can undergo 24-hour impedance-pH testing and consideration of antireflux surgery if ongoing GERD is demonstrated or they may remain on maximal medical therapy (**Fig. 4**). Additional studies directly comparing the 2 therapies will be useful to better establish the appropriate role of antireflux surgery in the management of difficult-to-eradicate intestinal metaplasia and dysplasia. With questions about the long-term effects of PPI therapy on cardiac, renal, and mental health, larger comparisons between PPI therapy and surgical antireflux surgery are interesting if they demonstrate equivalence or a potential medication-sparing effect in the longitudinal management of these patients.

SUMMARY

ER for the management of HGD and early mucosal cancers of the esophagus provides significant benefits compared with radical esophagectomy. EMR and ESD provide similar oncologic benefit via a less morbid and less invasive approach that precisely addresses the degree of the pathologic condition in these patients. Future studies are needed to better define the differences and relative benefits between EMR and ESD; specifically, the importance of the en bloc resection provided by ESD in the context of effective surveillance and ablative therapies partnered with EMR. As experience with ESD in the West increases and techniques such as tunneled ESD gain acceptance, the ease and efficiency of EMR may become less meaningful.

With endoscopic management as the first-line therapy for HGD and early esophageal cancers, it is important that esophageal and thoracic surgeons continue to play a direct and involved role in the diagnosis and treatment of these patients. Facility with EMR or ESD provides a strong continuity of care in the management of early esophageal malignancy from diagnosis, through early management and surgical resection if necessary. Familiarity with the advances in ER techniques also places thoracic surgeons in an ideal position to perform and guide additional research in this area to improve the quality of practice.

REFERENCES

1. Rice TW, Zuccaro G, Adelstein DJ, et al. Esophageal carcinoma: depth of tumor invasion is predictive of regional lymph node status. Ann Thorac Surg 1998;65(3):787–92.

2. Rice TW, Falk GW, Achkar E, et al. Surgical management of high-grade dysplasia in Barrett's esophagus. Am J Gastroenterol 1993;88:1832–6.

3. Ell C, May A, Pech O, et al. Curative endoscopic resection of early esophageal adenocarcinomas (Barrett's cancer). Gastrointest Endosc 2007; 65(1):3–10.

4. Shaheen NJ, Falk GW, Iyer PG, et al. ACG clinical guideline: diagnosis and management of Barrett's esophagus. Am J Gastroenterol 2016;111(1):30–50.

5. Ancona E, Rampado S, Cassaro M, et al. Prediction of lymph node status in superficial esophageal carcinoma. Ann Surg Oncol 2008;15(11):3278–88.

6. Griffin SM, Burt AD, Jennings NA. Lymph node metastasis in early esophageal adenocarcinoma. Ann Surg 2011;254(5):731–7.

7. Hölscher AH, Bollschweiler E, Schröder W, et al. Prognostic impact of upper, middle, and lower third mucosal or submucosal infiltration in early esophageal cancer. Ann Surg 2011;254:802–8.

8. Leers JM, DeMeester SR, Oezcelik A, et al. The prevalence of lymph node metastases in patients with T1 esophageal adenocarcinoma. Ann Surg 2011;253(2):271–8.

9. Pimentel-nunes P, Ponchon T, Repici A, et al. Endoscopic submucosal dissection: European Society of Gastrointestinal Endoscopy (ESGE) Guideline. Endoscopy 2015;47(9):829–54.

10. Ning B, Abdelfatah MM, Othma MO. Endoscopic submucosal dissection and endoscopic mucosal resection for early stage esophageal cancer. Ann Cardiothorac Surg 2017;6(2):88–98.

11. Kothari S, Kaul V. Endoscopic mucosal resection and endoscopic submucosal dissection for endoscopic therapy of Barrett's esophagus-related neoplasia. Gastroenterol Clin North Am 2015;44(2):317–35.

12. Koike T, Nakagawa K, Iijima K, et al. Endoscopic resection (endoscopic submucosal dissection/endoscopic mucosal resection) for superficial Barrett's esophageal cancer. Dig Endosc 2013; 25(Suppl.1):20–8.

13. Inoue H, Endo M. Endoscopic esophageal mucosal resection using a transparent tube. Surg Endosc 1990;4(4):198–201.

14. Pouw RE, Van Vilsteren FGI, Peters FP, et al. Randomized trial on endoscopic resection-cap versus multiband mucosectomy for piecemeal endoscopic resection of early Barrett's neoplasia. Gastrointest Endosc 2011;74(1):35–43.

15. Pech O, Behrens A, May A, et al. Long-term results and risk factor analysis for recurrence after curative endoscopic therapy in 349 patients with high-grade intraepithelial neoplasia and mucosal adenocarcinoma in Barrett's oesophagus. Gut 2008;57(9): 1200–6.

16. Pech O, May A, Manner H, et al. Long-term efficacy and safety of endoscopic resection for patients with mucosal adenocarcinoma of the esophagus. Gastroenterology 2014;146(3):652–60.e1.

17. Konda VJA, Gonzalez Haba Ruiz M, Koons A, et al. Complete endoscopic mucosal resection is effective and durable treatment for barrett's-associated neoplasia. Clin Gastroenterol Hepatol 2014;12(12): 2002–10.

18. May A, Gossner L, Pech O, et al. Local endoscopic therapy for intraepithelial high-grade neoplasia and early adenocarcinoma in Barrett's oesophagus: acute-phase and intermediate results of a new treatment approach. Eur J Gastroenterol Hepatol 2002; 14:1085–91.

19. Oliphant Z, Snow A, Knight H, et al. Endoscopic resection with or without mucosal ablation of high grade dysplasia and early oesophageal adenocarcinoma - long term follow up from a regional UK centre. Int J Surg 2014;12(11):1148–50.

20. Chadwick G, Groene O, Markar SR, et al. Systematic review comparing radiofrequency ablation and complete endoscopic resection in treating dysplastic Barrett's esophagus: a critical assessment of histologic outcomes and adverse events. Gastrointest Endosc 2014;79(5):718–31.e3.

21. Desai M, Saligram S, Gupta N, et al. Efficacy and safety outcomes of multimodal endoscopic eradication therapy in Barrett's esophagus-related neoplasia: a systematic review and pooled analysis. Gastrointest Endosc 2017;85(3):482–95.e4.

22. Guarner-Argente C, Buoncristiano T, Furth EE, et al. Long-term outcomes of patients with Barrett's esophagus and high-grade dysplasia or early cancer treated with endoluminal therapies with intention to complete eradication. Gastrointest Endosc 2013; 77(2):190–9.

23. Bhatt A, Abe S, Kumaravel A, et al. Indications and techniques for endoscopic submucosal dissection. Am J Gastroenterol 2015;110(6):784–91.

24. Pioche M, Mais L, Guillaud O, et al. Endoscopic submucosal tunnel dissection for large esophageal neoplastic lesions. Endoscopy 2013;45(12): 1032–4.

25. Zhai YQ, Li HK, Linghu EQ. Endoscopic submucosal tunnel dissection for large superficial esophageal squamous cell neoplasms. World J Gastroenterol 2016;22(1):435–45.

26. Joo DC, Kim GH, Park DY, et al. Long-term outcome after endoscopic submucosal dissection in patients with superficial esophageal squamous cell carcinoma: a single-center study. Gut Liver 2014;8(6): 612–8.

27. Yang D, Coman RM, Kahaleh M, et al. Endoscopic submucosal dissection for Barrett's early neoplasia: a multicenter study in the United States. Gastrointest Endosc 2016;86(4):600–7.

28. Subramaniam S, Chedgy F, Longcroft-Wheaton G, et al. Complex early Barrett's neoplasia at 3 Western centers: European Barrett's Endoscopic Submucosal Dissection Trial (E-BEST). Gastrointest Endosc 2017;86(4):608–18.

29. Coman RM, Gotoda T, Forsmark CE, et al. Prospective evaluation of the clinical utility of endoscopic submucosal dissection (ESD) in patients with Barrett's esophagus: a Western center experience. Endosc Int Open 2016;4(6):E715–21.

30. Takahashi H, Arimura Y, Masao H, et al. Endoscopic submucosal dissection is superior to conventional endoscopic resection as a curative treatment for early squamous cell carcinoma of the esophagus (with video). Gastrointest Endosc 2010;72(2):255–64.e2.

31. Guo H-M. Endoscopic submucosal dissection vs endoscopic mucosal resection for superficial esophageal cancer. World J Gastroenterol 2014;20(18):5540.

32. Park HC, Kim DH, Gong EJ, et al. Ten-year experience of esophageal endoscopic submucosal dissection of superficial esophageal neoplasms in a single center. Korean J Intern Med 2016;31(6): 1064–72.

33. Jin XF, Chai TH, Gai W, et al. Multiband mucosectomy versus endoscopic submucosal dissection for treatment of squamous intraepithelial neoplasia of the esophagus. Clin Gastroenterol Hepatol 2016; 14(7):948–55.

34. Chen Z, Ren Y, Du XL, et al. Incidence and survival differences in esophageal cancer among ethnic groups in the United States. Oncotarget 2017; 8(29):47037–51.

35. Huang R, Cai H, Zhao X, et al. Efficacy and safety of endoscopic submucosal tunnel dissection for superficial esophageal squamous cell carcinoma: a propensity score matching analysis. Gastrointest Endosc 2017;86(5):831–8.

36. Terheggen G, Horn EM, Vieth M, et al. A randomised trial of endoscopic submucosal dissection versus endoscopic mucosal resection for early Barrett's neoplasia. Gut 2017;66(5):783–93.

37. Yang D, Zou F, Xiong S, et al. Endoscopic submucosal dissection for early Barrett's neoplasia: a meta-analysis. Gastrointest Endosc 2017;1–11. https://doi.org/10.1016/j.gie.2017.09.038.

38. Park CH, Kim EH, Kim HY, et al. Clinical outcomes of endoscopic submucosal dissection for early stage esophagogastric junction cancer: a systematic review and meta-analysis. Dig Liver Dis 2015;47(1):37–44.

39. Pech O, Bollschweiler E, Manner H, et al. Comparison between endoscopic and surgical resection of mucosal esophageal adenocarcinoma in Barrett's esophagus at two high-volume centers. Ann Surg 2011;254(1):67–72.

40. Prasad GA, Wu TT, Wigle DA, et al. Endoscopic and surgical treatment of mucosal (T1a) esophageal

adenocarcinoma in Barrett's esophagus. Gastroenterology 2009;137(3):815–23.

41. Schembre DB, Huang JL, Lin OS, et al. Treatment of Barrett's esophagus with early neoplasia: a comparison of endoscopic therapy and esophagectomy. Gastrointest Endosc 2008;67(4):595–601.

42. Schmidt HM, Mohiuddin K, Bodnar AM, et al. Multidisciplinary treatment of T1a adenocarcinoma in Barrett's esophagus: contemporary comparison of endoscopic and surgical treatment in physiologically fit patients. Surg Endosc 2016;30(8): 3391–401.

43. McLaren PJ, Dolan JP. Esophagectomy as a treatment consideration for early-stage esophageal cancer and high-grade dysplasia. J Laparoendosc Adv Surg Tech A 2016;26(10):757–62.

44. Maish MS, DeMeester SR. Endoscopic mucosal resection as a staging technique to determine the depth of invasion of esophageal adenocarcinoma. Ann Thorac Surg 2004;78(5):1777–82.

45. Taioli E, Schwartz RM, Lieberman-Cribbin W, et al. Quality of life after open or minimally invasive esophagectomy in patients with esophageal cancer—a systematic review. Semin Thorac Cardiovasc Surg 2017;29(3):377–90.

46. Gupta M, Iyer PG, Lutzke L, et al. Recurrence of esophageal intestinal metaplasia after endoscopic mucosal resection and radiofrequency ablation of Barrett's esophagus: results from a US multicenter consortium. Gastroenterology 2013;145(1):79–86.e1.

47. Dubecz A, Kern M, Solymosi N, et al. Predictors of lymph node metastasis in surgically resected T1 esophageal cancer. Ann Thorac Surg 2015;99(6): 1879–86.

48. Boys JA, Worrell SG, Chandrasoma P, et al. Can the risk of lymph node metastases be gauged in endoscopically resected submucosal esophageal adenocarcinomas? A multi-center study. J Gastrointest Surg 2016;20(1):6–12.

49. Worrell SG, Boys JA, Chandrasoma P, et al. Interobserver variability in the interpretation of endoscopic mucosal resection specimens of esophageal adenocarcinoma: interpretation of ER specimens. J Gastrointest Surg 2016;20(1):140–5.

50. Parrilla P, Martinez de Haro LF, Ortiz A, et al. Long-term results of a randomized prospective study comparing medical and surgical treatment of Barrett's esophagus. Ann Surg 2003;237(3):291–8.

51. Oh DS, DeMeester SR, Vallbohmer D, et al. Reduction of interleukin 8 gene expression in reflux esophagitis and Barrett's esophagus with antireflux surgery. Arch Surg 2007;142(6):554–9.

52. Shimizu D, Vallböhmer D, Kuramochi H, et al. Increasing cyclooxygenase-2 (cox-2) gene expression in the progression of Barrett's esophagus to adenocarcinoma correlates with that of Bcl-2. Int J Cancer 2006;119(4):765–70.

53. O'Connell K, Velanovich V. Effects of Nissen fundoplication on endoscopic endoluminal radiofrequency ablation of Barrett's esophagus. Surg Endosc 2011;25(3):830–4.

54. Johnson CS, Louie BE, Wille A, et al. The durability of endoscopic therapy for treatment of Barrett's metaplasia, dysplasia, and mucosal cancer after Nissen fundoplication. J Gastrointest Surg 2015; 19(5):799–805.

55. Bulsiewicz WJ, Dellon ES, Lyday WD, et al. Predictors of recurrent barrett's esophagus after successful radiofrequency ablation in a nationwide, multicenter cohort: results from the U.S. RFA registry. Gastroenterology 2013;1(5):S1.

56. Skrobić O, Simić A, Radovanović N, et al. Significance of Nissen fundoplication after endoscopic radiofrequency ablation of Barrett's esophagus. Surg Endosc 2016;30(9):3802–7.

57. Komanduri S, Kahrilas PJ, Krishnan K, et al. Recurrence of Barrett's esophagus is rare following endoscopic eradication therapy coupled with effective reflux control. Am J Gastroenterol 2017;112(4):556–66.

Peroral Endoscopic Myotomy for Achalasia

Lara W. Schaheen, MD, Manuel Villa Sanchez, MD, James D. Luketich, MD*

KEYWORDS

- Achalasia • Peroral endoscopic myotomy (POEM) • Natural orifice surgery • Heller myotomy
- Minimally invasive • Dysphagia

KEY POINTS

- Achalasia is an uncommon disorder that requires careful evaluation.
- There are treatment options for achalasia that have variable efficacy.
- Peroral endoscopic myotomy is a rapidly emerging viable option for patients as a low-morbidity alternative to laparoscopic Heller myotomy.

INTRODUCTION

Achalasia is an acquired neurodegenerative disorder of the esophagus characterized by the failure of relaxation of the lower esophageal sphincter (LES) and presence of ineffective or absent peristalsis in the distal esophagus. Achalasia results from progressive degeneration of ganglion cells in the myenteric plexus in the esophageal wall. Degeneration of the intramuscular neural plexus leads to progressive loss of esophageal smooth muscle motility and failure of the LES's ability to relax receptively to peristalsis. This neuromotor degeneration is manifested most commonly by solid food dysphagia and progressively by vomiting or, more accurately, regurgitation of substances stuck in the esophagus. The failure of relaxation of the LES prevents food contents from emptying into the stomach, leading to a heartburnlike sensation, chest pain, and aspiration. The treatment of achalasia is aimed at decreasing the resting pressure in the LES to improve passage of ingested material, thereby improving quality of life and potentially preventing the complications related to this disease process.

EPIDEMIOLOGY

Achalasia is an uncommon disorder with an annual incidence of approximately 1.6 cases per 100,000 individuals and prevalence of 10 cases per 100,000 individuals.[1] Men and women are affected with equal frequency. The disease can occur at any age, but onset before adolescence is rare. Achalasia is usually diagnosed in patients between the ages of 25 and 60 years.

It may occur in association with adrenal insufficiency and alacrima in patients with triple A syndrome or Allgrove syndrome, a rare autosomal recessive genetic disorder.[2,3]

Etiology

The cause of primary or idiopathic achalasia is unknown. Secondary achalasia is due to diseases that cause esophageal motor abnormalities similar or identical to those of primary achalasia. In Chagas disease, an esophageal infection with the protozoan parasite *Trypanosoma cruzi*, which occurs predominantly in Central and South America, can result in a loss of intramural ganglion cells, leading to aperistalsis and incomplete LES relaxation.[4]

Disclosure: Dr L.W. Schaheen has nothing to disclose. Dr J.D. owns stock in Johnson & Johnson and Intuitive Surgical, Inc.
Department of Cardiothoracic Surgery, University of Pittsburgh Medical Center, UPMC Presbyterian, Suite C-800, 200 Lothrop Street, Pittsburgh, PA 15213, USA
* Corresponding author.
E-mail address: luketichjd@upmc.edu

Thorac Surg Clin 28 (2018) 499–506
https://doi.org/10.1016/j.thorsurg.2018.07.005
1547-4127/18/© 2018 Elsevier Inc. All rights reserved.

Other diseases that have been associated with achalasialike motor abnormalities include amyloidosis, sarcoidosis, neurofibromatosis, eosinophilic esophagitis, multiple endocrine neoplasia type 2B, juvenile Sjögren syndrome, chronic idiopathic intestinal pseudoobstruction, and Fabry disease.[5–11]

Pathogenesis

The cause of the inflammatory degeneration of neurons in primary achalasia is not known.[12] The observations that achalasia is associated with variants in the HLA-DQ region and that affected patients often have circulating antibodies to enteric neurons suggest that achalasia is an autoimmune disorder.[13–15] Some investigators have proposed that the inflammatory attack on esophageal neurons in achalasia is triggered by an antibody response to viral infections (eg, herpes zoster, measles viruses), but data have been inconclusive.[16,17]

PRESENTATION

The symptoms of achalasia are frequently misdiagnosed as heartburn/gastroesophageal reflux disease, esophageal strictures, or, sometimes, cardiac angina. Diagnosis of achalasia is frequently suggested by a barium swallow radiograph demonstrating varying degrees of dilation of the esophagus, narrowing at the level of the gastroesophageal sphincter and slow clearance of contents.[18] Definitive diagnosis and classification of the type of achalasia are made only with esophageal manometry.

On upper endoscopy, findings can include the classic "pop" on traversing the nonrelaxing LES, salivary stasis, and presence of residual food contents. Although upper endoscopy is not necessary to obtain a definitive diagnosis, it remains an important and necessary part of the diagnostic evaluation, as infiltrative adenocarcinoma of the LES is a cause of pseudoachalasia. Upper endoscopy affords the ability to evaluate and rule out other foregut pathology, such as stasis esophagitis and rarely squamous cell carcinoma.

Treatment

Treatment of achalasia is aimed at decreasing the resting pressure in the LES to facilitate the passage of ingested material into the stomach. Unfortunately, no treatment can reverse the degeneration of ganglion cells and normalize esophageal function. Consequently, currently available treatments merely aim to manage or improve symptoms.

Surgical myotomy has been the most reliable treatment of choice for treating esophageal achalasia since the first report by Heller in 1913.[19] Laparoscopic surgery (Heller myotomy and partial fundoplication) has the highest efficacy and long-term success rates (90%–95% relief of dysphagia, persisting >10 years for 85% of patients).[20]

Other management methods include pharmacologic with smooth muscle relaxants, and calcium channel blockers, balloon dilatation, and botulinum toxin injection.[21] All of the currently effective invasive treatment options are aimed at mechanical disruption of the muscle fibers of the LES (eg, pneumatic dilation, surgical myotomy or peroral endoscopic myotomy) or by pharmacologic reduction in LES pressure (eg, injection of botulinum toxin).

Development of Peroral Endoscopic Myotomy

The idea of incisionless endoscopic treatment options for achalasia first began with Ortega and colleagues[22] in the 1980s when they used an electrosurgical knife to perform an endoscopic transmucosal myotomy in dogs. But because of concerns for the mediastinal contamination inherent in the creation of a full-thickness esophageal incision, the technique failed to gain momentum. Over the course of the next 30 years, several important innovations would lead to a renewed interest in the endoscopic myotomy technique. It was the understanding that the submucosal space could be used to access the muscular layer of the esophagus that led to the development of a submucosal tunneling technique.[23] Furthermore, by offsetting the site of mucosal entry from the beginning of the myotomy, a mucosal flap would be created, which allowed for further protection from mediastinal contamination.[24] In 2010, Haruhiro Inoue introduced peroral endoscopic myotomy in humans as an endoscopic treatment for esophageal achalasia. Inoue and colleagues[25] further refined the peroral endoscopic myotomy surgery (POEMS) technique by dividing the circular muscle layer of the LES and leaving the longitudinal muscle layer intact.

Since its introduction, POEMS has been rapidly developing into one of the standard treatments for esophageal achalasia and related esophageal motility diseases, such as diffuse esophageal spasm and jackhammer esophagus.[25–27] The excitement that POEM has engendered is because it offers the efficacy of surgery with the cost and morbidity of a purely endoscopic procedure.

SURGICAL TECHNIQUE
Patient Selection

POEM is indicated for all patients with symptomatic achalasia. There are few contraindications to POEM outside of comorbid conditions preventing general endotracheal anesthesia.[25,28] Relative contraindications include prior history of esophageal submucosal resection, prior radiation to the mediastinum, severe pulmonary disease, cirrhosis with portal hypertension, and inability to safely stop systemic anticoagulation.[29]

Preoperative Planning

The patient who presents to the authors' clinic with dysphagia or other foregut complaints undergoes a series of routine tests that include the following:

1. Detailed history and physical examination
2. Routine laboratory work including nutritional laboratories
3. Chest radiograph
4. Timed barium esophagram
5. Esophageal manometry
6. Upper endoscopy
7. Chest and abdominal computed tomography (selective)
8. Gastric emptying study (selective)

Esophagogastroduodenoscopy (EGD), barium swallow, and manometry should be performed preoperatively in all patients. Upper endoscopy provides important information regarding the severity of esophageal dilation and tortuosity, degree of underlying esophagitis, and presence of potential esophageal malignancy. Barium esophagram provides important information about the dynamics of the esophagus, such as the presence or absence of peristaltic contractions, and serves as a roadmap of the esophageal anatomy. Esophageal manometry is an essential diagnostic tool for the evaluation of detailed esophageal function and the confirmation of the diagnosis.

Once the preoperative testing has been completed and the diagnosis of achalasia confirmed, the patient undergoes an informed consent discussion regarding the available treatment options. Patient age, symptoms, and esophageal anatomy are important considerations in planning and targeting what will be the most effective therapy for them. It is not uncommon for patients to choose the least invasive options before proceeding to a more invasive treatment. Of note, a history of prior endoscopic treatment does not preclude patients from receiving a POEM, laparoscopic Heller myotomy, or rarely esophagectomy.

Prep and Patient Positioning

In preparation for the POEM procedure, patients are placed on a full liquid diet for 3 days before the procedure.[30] On the day before undergoing the procedure patients are further restricted to a clear liquid diet. In patients with a tortuous or significantly dilated esophagus, an additional 3 days of a clear liquid diet is added to ensure an empty esophagus on the day of the procedure. The patient is placed in the supine position on the operating room table. General anesthesia and endotracheal intubation are performed with the assumption that the esophagus may still be full of old food and debris. It is essential that the surgeon be present during intubation and assist in performing the Sellick maneuver to minimize the risk of aspiration of esophageal contents. Broad-spectrum intravenous antibiotics are administered before initiation of the procedure. EGD is then performed in order to clear the esophagus of any residual food contents. At the initiation of endoscopy the starting peak airway pressures are confirmed with the anesthesiologist. The patient's abdomen remains exposed during the procedure in order to allow for evaluation for captoperitoneum.

SURGICAL PROCEDURE

The peroral endoscopic myotomy is performed using a forward-viewing high-definition endoscope with a transparent cap attached distally. Continuous carbon dioxide (CO_2) insufflation at a constant rate of 1.2 L/min is used to allow for improved visualization and creation of the submucosal plane. An overtube is advanced into the esophagus and secured in place. The esophagus is then evaluated and distance to the LES measured.

The conduct of the POEM operation is stepwise as follows[28–31]:

1. Mucosal incision
2. Creation of a submucosal tunnel
3. Myotomy
4. Closure of mucosal incision

The details of each step are as follows:

Mucosal Incision

The site of mucosal incision should be approximately 10 to 12 cm proximal to the measured gastroesophageal junction. Approximately 10 mL of normal saline supplemented with dilute methylene blue is injected into the submucosal space on the anterior (12 o'clock) position of the midesophagus. The injection of the methylene blue saline solution should create a wheal under the mucosa. Using an endoscopic knife, a 2-cm longitudinal mucosal incision is made on the previously created mucosal wheal. Using a combination of CO_2 insufflation and electrocautery, the areolar tissue of the submucosal space is dissected until the circular muscle layers are identified. Once an adequate mucosal flap is created the endoscope with the translucent cap is inserted into the submucosal space (**Fig. 1**).

Creation of the Submucosal Tunnel

Once inside the submucosal space the endoscope is oriented to maintain the mucosa at the 6 o'clock position and circular muscle fibers at the 12 o'clock position. The submucosal tunnel should be continued 2 to 3 cm beyond the gastroesophageal junction and onto the proximal stomach (**Fig. 2**). In order to allow for easy manipulation of the endoscope, the tunnel should be widened to approximately one-third of the esophageal circumference. Periodically, it may be necessary to exit the submucosal tunnel and enter the native lumen of the esophagus to decompress the stomach. Overdistension of the stomach can be avoided by maintaining visualization of the abdominal wall and an ongoing dialogue with anesthesia regarding blood pressure, airway pressure, and end-tidal CO_2. If there are any significant concerns, the first step should be to enter the native lumen and evacuate the stomach. If problems persist, placement of an intrathoracic pigtail catheter or varices needle decompression of the abdomen should be considered.

The gastroesophageal junction can be identified by a change of the vascular pattern and palisade vessels or use of a double scope technique in

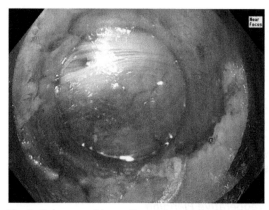

Fig. 2. Submucosal tunneling. A long submucosal tunnel is created and carried 2 to 3 cm distal to the gastroesophageal junction. The circular muscle fibers are perpendicular to the longitudinal direction of the tunnel.

which a second endoscope is used to obtain a retroflexed view of the gastric cardia, whereas the dissecting scope trans illuminates from the end of the submucosal tunnel.

Myotomy

Dissection of the circular muscle fibers should begin 3 to 4 cm distal from the mucosal entry site (**Fig. 3**). The circular muscle fibers are divided while preserving the integrity of the longitudinal muscle fibers. The coagulation current of the endoscopic knife is used in order to avoid bleeding from the intramuscular vessels. Division of the muscle fibers should be continued for 2 to 3 cm onto the gastric cardia. In order to determine if

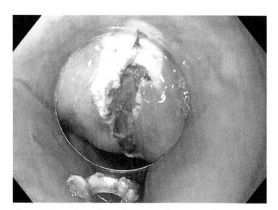

Fig. 1. Entry into the submucosal space. After submucosal injection of saline and dilute methylene blue dye, a 2-cm longitudinal mucosal incision is made at the midesophagus.

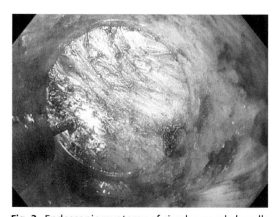

Fig. 3. Endoscopic myotomy of circular muscle bundle begins from 4 to 5 cm distal to the mucosal entry and extends to 2 to 3 cm distal to the gastroesophageal junction. By using a triangle tip knife, endoscopic myotomy of inner circular muscle bundles is done, leaving the outer longitudinal muscle layer intact.

your circular muscle division is adequate, one can return the scope to the native esophageal lumen and assess for residual narrowing at the level of the gastroesophageal junction.

Closure of the Mucosal Incision

Before closure of the mucosal incision the submucosal tunnel is irrigated copiously with antibiotic solution. The mucosal incision is closed with hemostatic clips. The first clip is placed just beyond the most distal aspect of the mucosal incision in order to create a mucosal fold or ridge. The translucent cap of the endoscope can be used to apply downward pressure on the clip in order to evert the mucosal edges and make clip application easier. Complete closure of the mucosal incision is confirmed endoscopically (**Fig. 4**). If there are concerns that the closure is not adequate, placement of a covered esophageal stent may be considered. In the first 30 cases, the authors placed a stent in 2 cases due to these concerns with good results.[32]

POSTOPERATIVE CARE

Patients are admitted to the monitored surgical floor postoperatively and allowed sips of water following recovery from general anesthesia. An esophagram with water-soluble contrast is performed on the morning of postoperative day 1 to evaluate for leak. Patients are maintained on a clear liquid diet until postoperative day 3 when a full liquid diet is started. Patients continue a full liquid diet until postoperative day 5 in which time they are transitioned to a soft diet until outpatient follow-up. Patients are observed in the hospital until it is confirmed that an oral diet is tolerated and that there is no clinical evidence of a delayed leak. At the time of discharge, patients are carefully instructed to call the authors' office immediately should any signs of systemic illness occur. Patients are seen in clinic for routine follow-up in 2 weeks. At 12 months from POEM, patients undergo a barium esophagram and comprehensive symptom assessment.

CLINICAL RESULTS IN THE LITERATURE

POEM has been demonstrated to be a safe and feasible intervention capable of significantly improving dysphagia and a patient's ability to eat. In most clinical series, pre- and post-POEM Eckhardt scores are used as a measure of treatment efficacy and define clinical success as a post-POEM Eckhardt score less than 3. Early series reported the clinical success of POEM to be 82% to 100% at 12 months, many reporting greater than 90% improvement in symptoms. However, it should be noted that many of the early series published had a relatively short follow-up period. Inoue reported the outcomes of 500 consecutive patients treated with POEMS with a follow-up of more than 3 years. This study showed that 2-month, 1- to 2-year, and 3-year overall success rates were 91.3%, 91.0%, and 88.5%, respectively.[29] In comparison with laparoscopic Heller myotomy with or without fundoplication, POEM has demonstrated similar relief of dysphagia as evidenced by decreased Eckardt scores and decreased resting pressures of the LES.[33–37]

One of the concerns as the POEM procedure gained popularity was the absence of a partial fundoplication to provide a reflux barrier. Initial series reported an incidence of symptomatic GERD from 0% to 37% but was thought to be controlled with a single dose of proton pump inhibitors (PPI).[29] More recent studies have demonstrated that the development of reflux and PPI use does not seem to be significantly different between laparoscopic Heller myotomy and POEM.[34,36]

As previous intervention at the gastroesophageal junction may result in some degree of submucosal fibrosis, it was thought by some that prior intervention could make peroral endoscopic myotomy more difficult. Several retrospective studies have demonstrated that a history of prior intervention does not result in worse outcomes.[38–40] POEM has also been demonstrated to be successful in the setting of recurrence or failure after previous surgical myotomy. The results of 3 studies examining the utility of POEM in patients who have undergone a previous surgical myotomy have been published. Several recent series have examined outcomes in patients whose symptoms recurred after Heller myotomy and subsequently received a salvage POEM. These series showed

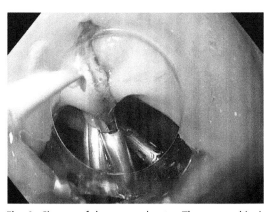

Fig. 4. Closure of the mucosal entry. The mucosal incision of entry point is completely closed with hemostatic clips.

acceptable feasibility, safety, and relatively high clinical efficacy in the range of 91.7% to 100%.[41,42]

Although more recent studies have demonstrated that POEM can be performed safely in patients who have undergone previous endoscopic intervention or surgery for achalasia, at the extremes of age (2 years to 90 years) and in the setting of end-stage achalasia with a mega or sigmoid esophagus the authors recommend a cautious approach when introducing this into clinical practice because unrecognized complications carry significant morbidity. In a large retrospective study published by Zhang and colleagues,[43] delayed mucosal closure occurred in 0.8%, delayed bleeding in 0.2%, hydrothorax requiring intervention in 0.5%, and pneumothorax requiring intervention in 1.5%.

The rapidly growing interest in POEM has lead to completion by a multiple types of interventionalists with a wide variety of skill sets. A recent single-center retrospective study published by El Zein and colleagues[44,45] aimed to define the learning curve for POEM. They found that an expert interventional endoscopist required a minimum of 13 cases before demonstrating a plateau in total operative time.

As the morbidity associated with an esophageal injury can be great, the authors believe the procedure should be performed in the operating room under the care of a surgeon with extensive experience in laparoscopic and open treatment of achalasia. In an effort to optimize early success, the authors suggest that surgeons participate in a hands-on course, observe an expert performing several POEM procedures, and perform their first few procedures on straightforward cases with an experienced proctor present. In our early experience at the University of Pittsburgh, the same surgeon and first assist performed the procedure with the assistance of a dedicated operating room team. The learning curve is significant and it is clear that even after 50 cases, the authors believe, these cases demand a high level of experience and caution throughout the procedure and an extremely vigilant and cautious postop course as well.

SUMMARY

Achalasia is an uncommon esophageal motility disorder that has significant effects on quality of life and is associated with significant morbidity if left untreated. Although there are multiple treatment options available, laparoscopic myotomy and partial fundoplication remains the gold standard by which all achalasia treatment modalities should be compared. POEM has gained widespread popularity because it offers an incisionless minimally invasive treatment to achalasia. Early experience has demonstrated that it provides symptomatic relief of dysphagia that is equivalent to that of laparoscopic Heller myotomy. Further studies are required to define the durability of relief of symptoms and long-term outcomes. POEM represents a paradigm shift for patients with achalasia and the results of long-term follow-up of randomized prospective trials are eagerly awaited.

REFERENCES

1. Sadowski DC, Ackah F, Jiang B, et al. Achalasia: incidence, prevalence and survival. A population-based study. Neurogastroenterol Motil 2010;22: e256.
2. Allgrove J, Clayden GS, Grant DB, et al. Familial glucocorticoid deficiency with achalasia of the cardia and deficient tear production. Lancet 1978; 1:1284.
3. Verma S, Brown S, Dakkak M, et al. Association of adult achalasia and alacrima. Dig Dis Sci 1999; 44:876.
4. De Oliveira RB, Rezende Filho J, Dantas RO, et al. The spectrum of esophageal motor disorders in Chagas' disease. Am J Gastroenterol 1995;90:1119.
5. Costigan DJ, Clouse RE. Achalasia-like esophagus from amyloidosis. Successful treatment with pneumatic bag dilation. Dig Dis Sci 1983;28:763.
6. Dufresne CR, Jeyasingham K, Baker RR. Achalasia of the cardia associated with pulmonary sarcoidosis. Surgery 1983;94:32.
7. Foster PN, Stewart M, Lowe JS, et al. Achalasia like disorder of the oesophagus in von Recklinghausen's neurofibromatosis. Gut 1987;28:1522.
8. Cuthbert JA, Gallagher ND, Turtle JR. Colonic and oesophageal disturbance in a patient with multiple endocrine neoplasia, type 2b. Aust N Z J Med 1978;8:518.
9. Similä S, Kokkonen J, Kaski M. Achalasia sicca–juvenile Sjögren's syndrome with achalasia and gastric hyposecretion. Eur J Pediatr 1978;129:175.
10. Schuffler MD. Chronic intestinal pseudo-obstruction syndromes. Med Clin North Am 1981;65:1331.
11. Roberts DH, Gilmore IT. Achalasia in Anderson-Fabry's disease. J R Soc Med 1984;77:430.
12. Kilic A, Krasinskas AM, Owens SR, et al. Variations in inflammation and nerve fiber loss reflect different subsets of achalasia patients. J Surg Res 2007; 143:177.
13. Wong RK, Maydonovitch CL, Metz SJ, et al. Significant DQw1 association in achalasia. Dig Dis Sci 1989;34:349.

14. Verne GN, Sallustio JE, Eaker EY. Anti-myenteric neuronal antibodies in patients with achalasia. A prospective study. Dig Dis Sci 1997;42:307.

15. Verne GN, Hahn AB, Pineau BC, et al. Association of HLA-DR and -DQ alleles with idiopathic achalasia. Gastroenterology 1999;117:26.

16. Niwamoto H, Okamoto E, Fujimoto J, et al. Are human herpes viruses or measles virus associated with esophageal achalasia? Dig Dis Sci 1995;40:859.

17. Birgisson S, Galinski MS, Goldblum JR, et al. Achalasis is not associated with measles or known herpes and human papilloma viruses. Dig Dis Sci 1997;42:300.

18. Eckardt VF. Clinical presentations and complications of achalasia. Gastrointest Endosc Clin N Am 2001; 11:281.

19. Heller E. Extramukose kardioplastik beim chronischen kardiospasm mit dilatation des oesophagus. Mitt Greenzgeb Med Chir 1913;27:141.

20. Richards WO, Torquati A, Holzman MD, et al. Heller myotomy versus Heller myotomy with Dor fundoplication for achalasia: a prospective randomized double-blind clinical trial. Ann Surg 2004;240:405–12.

21. Vaezi MF, Pandolfino JE, Vela MF. ACG clinical guideline: diagnosis and management of achalasia. Am J Gastroenterol 2013;108:1238.

22. Ortega JA, Madureri V, Perez L. Endoscopic myotomy in the treatment of achalasia. Gastrointest Endosc 1980;26:8–10.

23. Pasricha PJ, Hawari R, Ahmed I, et al. Submucosal endoscopic esophageal myotomy: a novel experimental approach for the treatment of achalasia. Endoscopy 2007;39:761–4.

24. Sumiyama K, Gostout CJ, Rajan E, et al. Submucosal endoscopy with mucosal flap safety valve. Gastrointest Endosc 2007;65:688–94.

25. Inoue H, Minami H, Kobayashi Y, et al. Peroral endoscopic myotomy (POEM) for esophageal achalasia. Endoscopy 2010;42:265–71.

26. Minami H, Isomoto H, Yamaguchi N, et al. Peroral endoscopic myotomy (POEM) for diffuse esophageal spasm. Endoscopy 2014;46:E79–81.

27. Shiwaku H, Inoue H, Beppu R, et al. Successful treatment of diffuse esophageal spasm by peroral endoscopic myotomy. Gastrointest Endosc 2013; 77:149–50.

28. Grimes KL, Inoue H. Per oral endoscopic myotomy for achalasia: a detailed description of the technique and review of the literature. Thorac Surg Clin 2016; 26:147–62.

29. Inoue H, Sato H, Ikeda H, et al. Per-oral endoscopic myotomy: a series of 500 patients. J Am Coll Surg 2015;221:256–64.

30. Stavropoulos SN, Modayil RJ, Friedel D, et al. The international per oral endoscopic myotomy survey (IPOEMS): a snapshot of the global POEM experience. Surg Endosc 2013;27:3322.

31. Swanström LL, Rieder E, Dunst CM. A stepwise approach and early clinical experience in peroral endoscopic myotomy for the treatment of achalasia and esophageal motility disorders. J Am Coll Surg 2011;213:751–6.

32. Schaheen LW, Odell DD, Chan EG, et al. Preliminary experience with per-oral endoscopic myotomy (poems) by a thoracic surgical service. Proceedings of the American Association for Thoracic Surgery 96th Annual Meeting, Baltimore, MD, May 14–16, 2016. p. 158–9.

33. Hungness ES, Teitelbaum EN, Santos BF, et al. Comparison of perioperative outcomes between peroral esophageal myotomy (POEM) and laparoscopic Heller myotomy. J Gastrointest Surg 2013; 17:228–35.

34. Bhayani NH, Kurian AA, Dunst CM, et al. A comparative study on comprehensive, objective outcomes of laparoscopic Heller myotomy with per-oral endoscopic myotomy (POEM) for achalasia. Ann Surg 2014;259:1098–103.

35. Sanaka MR, Hayat U, Thota PN, et al. Efficacy of peroral endoscopic myotomy vs other achalasia treatments in improving esophageal function. World J Gastroenterol 2016;22:4918–25.

36. Schneider AM, Louie BE, Warren HF, et al. A matched comparison of per oral endoscopic myotomy to laparoscopic heller myotomy in the treatment of achalasia. J Gastrointest Surg 2016;20:1789–96.

37. Peng L, Tian S, Du C, et al. Outcome of peroral endoscopic myotomy (POEM) for Treating Achalasia Compared With Laparoscopic Heller Myotomy (LHM). Surg Laparosc Endosc Percutan Tech 2017;27:60–4.

38. Sharata A, Kurian AA, Dunst CM, et al. Peroral endoscopic myotomy (POEM) is safe and effective in the setting of prior endoscopic intervention. J Gastrointest Surg 2013;17:1188–92.

39. Orenstein SB, Raigani S, Wu YV, et al. Peroral endoscopic myotomy (POEM) leads to similar results in patients with and without prior endoscopic or surgical therapy. Surg Endosc 2015;29:1064–70.

40. Jones EL, Meara MP, Pittman MR, et al. Prior treatment does not influence the performance or early outcome of per-oral endoscopic myotomy for achalasia. Surg Endosc 2016;30:1282–6.

41. Zhou PH, Li QL, Yao LQ, et al. Peroral endoscopic remyotomy for failed Heller myotomy: a prospective single-center study. Endoscopy 2013;45:161–6.

42. Onimaru M, Inoue H, Ikeda H, et al. Peroral endoscopic myotomy is a viable option for failed surgical esophagocardiomyotomy instead of redo surgical Heller myotomy: a single center prospective study. J Am Coll Surg 2013;217:598–605.

43. Zhang XC, Li QL, Xu MD, et al. Major perioperative adverse events of peroral endoscopic myotomy: a systematic 5-year analysis. Endoscopy 2016;48: 967–78.

44. Hungness ES, Sternbach JM, Teitelbaum EN, et al. Per-oral endoscopic myotomy (POEM) after the learning curve: durable long-term results with a low complication rate. Ann Surg 2016;264: 508.

45. El Zein M, Kumbhari V, Ngamruengphong S, et al. Learning curve for peroral endoscopic myotomy. Endosc Int Open 2016;4(5):E577–82.

Endoscopic Approaches to Cricopharyngeal Myotomy and Pyloromyotomy

Anee Sophia Jackson, MD[a], Ralph W. Aye, MD[b],*

KEYWORDS

• Endoscopic cricopharyngeal myotomy • Zenker's diverticulum • Endoscopic pyloromyotomy

KEY POINTS

- Endoscopic cricopharyngeal myotomy is a safe and efficacious procedure in the treatment of cricopharyngeal dysfunction with or without Zenker's diverticulum.
- Flexible endoscopic approach in the treatment of Zenker's diverticulum is an evolving technique circumventing limitations presented in the rigid endoscopic approach.
- Peroral endoscopic pyloromyotomy is a novel technique for the management of gastroparesis with promising outcomes in early studies.

This article describes the use of endoscopic techniques to address dysfunction at the entrance to the esophagus, the upper esophageal sphincter, and at the exit of the stomach, the pylorus. The authors introduce a brief anatomy and workup for patients with a hypertonic cricopharyngeus (CP) muscle with or without a Zenker's diverticulum (ZD) and do the same for patients with gastroparesis requiring a pyloromyotomy. The novel techniques of both the endoscopic cricopharyngeal myotomy (CPM) and the endoscopic pyloromyotomy will be discussed in detail.

ENDOSCOPIC CRICOPHARYNGEAL MYOTOMY WITH AND WITHOUT ZENKER'S DIVERTICULUM
Introduction

The CP muscle is the main muscular structure of the upper esophageal sphincter (UES). The CP is a ring-shaped muscle composed of horizontal and oblique fibers and is under a steady state of contraction at rest providing luminal occlusion and preventing retrograde reflux entering the pharynx and antegrade air entering the esophagus.[1] During the normal physiologic swallowing process, the CP relaxes to open the cricopharyngeal region and allow the passage of the food bolus. Derangement of the CP can be due to multiple causes and can lead to a spectrum of symptoms from dysphagia to severe aspiration to development of ZD. There is no direct therapy to address an incompetent CP, and management of fibrotic stricture is a separate topic. This section focuses on surgical options for dysphagia/aspiration and ZD caused by hypercontractile or obstructing CP.

Anatomy

Understanding the physiology of swallowing and the anatomy of the UES, especially the fascial planes and potential spaces, is important in a successful endoscopic CPM as well as management of the potential complications. The UES is

Disclosure Statement: The authors have nothing to disclose.
[a] Division of Thoracic Surgery, Swedish Cancer Institute, 1101 Madison Street, Suite 900, Seattle, WA 98104, USA; [b] Thoracic Oncology, Advanced GI, Thoracic Fellowships, Division of Thoracic Surgery, Swedish Cancer Institute, 1101 Madison Street, Suite 900, Seattle, WA 98104, USA
* Corresponding author.
E-mail address: ralph.aye@swedish.org

composed of the inferior constrictor muscle, the CP muscle, and the upper part of the cervical esophagus. The CP is a ring-shaped muscle composed of horizontal and oblique fibers and is the main muscular structure of the UES (**Fig. 1**). During normal swallowing, inhibitory signals control the relaxation of the CP before the arrival of the advancing bolus. In addition, the larynx elevates and moves anteriorly to further open the CP. Once the bolus passes, the CP returns to its contracted state.[2] It is thought that pharyngoesophageal (Zenker's) diverticula occur due to a combination of increased hypopharyngeal pressure during swallowing and obstructive dysfunction of the CP leading to a herniation through the muscle layers in the weak area between the transverse fibers of the CP and the oblique fibers of the lower inferior constrictor muscles. This area of weakness is known as Killian's triangle.

The buccopharyngeal fascia surrounds the CP, esophagus, and inferior pharyngeal constrictors. It is the visceral component of the middle layer of the deep cervical fascia and runs from the skull base superiorly to the fibrous pericardium of the mediastinum inferiorly. Behind the buccopharyngeal fascia is the retropharyngeal space that is defined posteriorly by the alar fascia. Continuing posteriorly, the danger space lies behind the alar fascia. The danger space is from the skull base to diaphragm and is defined posteriorly by the prevertebral fascia.[3] The prevertebral space is posterior to the prevertebral fascia (**Fig. 2**). It is the violation of these fascial layers that can lead to rapidly spreading infection from pharyngeal contents.

Chang and colleagues[4] performed an anatomic study on cadavers while performing an endoscopic CPM with carbon dioxide (CO_2) laser. After the procedure was performed, the buccopharyngeal fascia remained intact protecting the retropharyngeal space. Even if the buccopharyngeal fascia was violated, the leaked pharyngeal contents were contained in the retropharyngeal areolar tissue. Both of these structures, the buccopharyngeal fascia and the areolar tissue in the retropharyngeal space, are violated with dissection in the open, transcervical approach. In endoscopic CPM, it is the preservation of these structures that minimize the risk of mediastinitis.[5]

Indications and Diagnosis

UES dysfunction causing oropharyngeal dysphagia can be due to multiple causes, including both central and peripheral neurologic disorders, myogenic disorders, iatrogenic injury from previous neck surgery or radiation, distal esophageal dysfunction such as gastroesophageal reflux, old age, or idiopathic. Patient complaints can range from a globus sensation to severe dysphagia with sticking of food and in more extreme cases, aspiration and other associated morbidities such as weight loss. Cricopharyngeal dysmotility can lead to ZD, the most common indication for CPM.[6] In patients with ZD, presenting symptoms can also include regurgitation of food, halitosis, and chronic cough in addition to dysphagia and aspiration associated with CP dysfunction alone.

Several causes are not amenable to CPM as a treatment for their oropharyngeal dysphagia. These include presence of tumor that involves the cervical esophagus, prior neck radiation because the fibrotic CP is less likely to separate when sectioned, and severe pharyngeal dysfunction from progressive neurologic disorders.[3] Another contraindication to endoscopic CPM includes trismus. With the use of the flexible endoscopic approach in treatment of CP dysfunction, cervical disease that prevents neck hyperextension is no longer a contraindication to endoscopic treatment.

A patient is a candidate for CPM based on a thorough history and workup to identify isolated dysfunction of the CP and explore the presence of ZD. Diagnostic imaging and procedures include video fluoroscopic swallow study, flexible endoscopy, manofluorography (manometry with

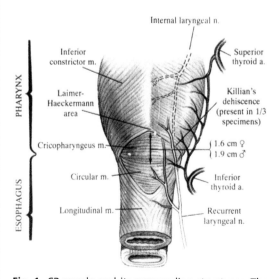

Fig. 1. CP muscle and its surrounding structures. The CP muscle is the main muscular structure of the upper esophageal sphincter. a, artery; m, muscle; n, nerve. (*From* Kelly JH. Management of upper esophageal sphincter disorders: indications and complications of myotomy. Am J Med 2000;108(Suppl 4a):44S; with permission.)

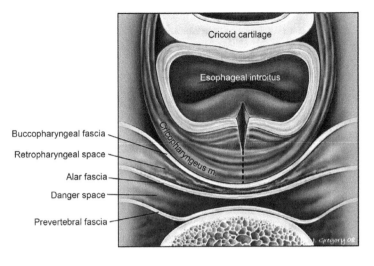

Fig. 2. CP muscle and surrounding fascial layers. (*From* Pitman MJ, Weissbrod P. Endoscopic CO_2 laser cricopharyngeal myotomy. Laryngoscope 2009;119:48; with permission.)

videofluorography), and electromyography. On a barium swallow study, the classic finding of failure of the CP to relax is the presence of a horizontal bar (cricopharyngeal bar) at the level of the cricoid cartilage. This bar makes a posterior indentation in the barium column that persists throughout the swallow.[3] This cricopharyngeal bar can also be seen on flexible endoscopy. It is also important to look for any tumor that could be causing the CP dysfunction during endoscopy. When a ZD is present, it can be seen on both swallow studies and endoscopy as a midline protrusion at the level of the posterior hypopharyngeal wall, just above the CP (**Fig. 3**). In addition, on endoscopy, a "dividing bar" or septum can be seen between the diverticulum and the true esophageal lumen (**Fig. 4**).[7]

Manometric tracings can reveal abnormalities in UES, including elevated resting pressure, elevated intrabolus pressure, as well as abnormalities in coordination.[8] Manofluorography is another tool for evaluation in which manometry is performed with videofluoroscopy. This allows for the correlation of anatomical structure during swallowing with intraluminal pressures, and a mid-intrabolus pressure gradient can be determined, which acts as an indirect measurement of UES compliance.[2,5,9] Video nasofiberoscopy and electromyography of the pharynx and CP can also be used in the workup.[10] Electromyography of the pharynx and CP allows for simultaneous recordings of the muscles and provides information on the myoelectric activity, such as lack of synchronism in contraction between the muscles, hyperactivity, and failure to relax.[11]

Balloon dilations and injection of botulinum toxin can be both diagnostic and therapeutic in isolated CP dysfunction. There are few small

series of patients receiving balloon catheter dilation as a treatment for cricopharyngeal dysphagia with successful improvement.[12,13] Many of the reported patients were elderly because balloon dilation may be an attractive option in elderly patients with many comorbidities. Injection of botulinum toxin can temporarily relieve dysphagia. Most reports of the use of botulinum toxin injections are described with administration under general anesthesia via direct laryngoscopy under endoscopic guidance, because adequate visualization and localization with flexible endoscopy can be challenging.[1,14] Transcutaneous injection

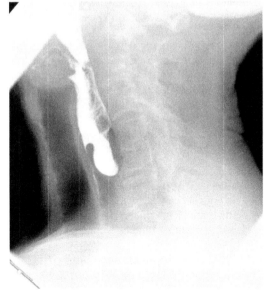

Fig. 3. A ZD can be seen as a midline protrusion at the level of the posterior hypopharyngeal wall on a swallow study.

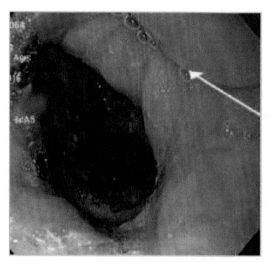

Fig. 4. An endoscopic view of a ZD with the arrow pointing to the esophageal opening. The septum/CP bar can be seen between the ZD and esophageal opening.

of botulinum toxin with local anesthesia without sedation has been reported. This office-based approach uses electromyography to guide the injection.[15,16] Complications reported after botulinum toxin injection are infrequent but can be serious, including a temporary worsening of dysphagia, neck cellulitis, transient vocal fold paralysis, and aspiration.[17] If a patient has a good response with improvement in dysphagia symptoms with the botulinum toxin injection, it is likely that myotomy also will help[14,18]; although, failure of botulinum toxin to improve symptoms does not mean that a patient will not respond well to CPM.[6]

There is no gold standard for the diagnosis of CP dysfunction, but based on a combination of the studies discussed earlier as well as a thorough history, treatment is indicated for patients identified with CP hypertonicity/obstruction ± ZD with preserved laryngeal swallowing and propulsion of food bolus. Factors that favor a successful surgical outcome include the following[19]:

- Intact swallowing initiation
- Adequate laryngeal/hyoid elevation
- Pharyngeal propulsion with swallowing
- Radiographic or manometric evidence of failed relaxation of the CP muscle

Technique: Endoscopic Management of Cricopharyngeal Myotomy Without Zenker's Diverticulum

Once obstructive CP dysfunction is diagnosed after a rigorous assessment, a variety of management approaches can be used, including dilation, intramuscular injection of botulinum toxin, and CPM. Although dilation and Botox can serve as both a diagnostic and therapeutic technique temporarily relieving dysphagia, CPM is the only method that can provide a definitive cure.[1,20–22] The traditional approach to CPM is through an open, left-sided, transcervical approach. Although the open approach is effective, it requires an open incision and includes risks such as hematoma, recurrent laryngeal nerve injury, pharyngocutaneous fistula, and infection to both the wound and, more seriously, the retropharyngeal space.[23,24]

In 1994, Halvorson and Kuhn described the first endoscopic technique for isolated CPM without ZD using direct laryngoscopy with a potassium titanyl phosphate laser to incise the CP.[25] Soon thereafter, the CO_2 laser gained popularity and is used widely today in the procedure.[5] Endoscopic CPM has been shown to be a safe and efficient alternative with shorter operative time, improved outcomes, and reduced scarring/stricture compared with the open approach.[10,26–29] However, studies that focus on endoscopic CPM are limited and relatively small in sample size with patients with multiple different etiologies, and the procedure remains a novel approach. The authors aim to describe the technique of the endoscopic CPM.

The patient is placed in a supine position, and the procedure is performed under general anesthesia. A diverticuloscope is placed as far as the esophageal inlet, postcricoid to obtain exposure. If needed, a nasogastric tube can be used to help guide the placement of the diverticuloscope by designating the esophageal inlet. By lifting the larynx with pressure from the diverticuloscope, the CP can be better visualized. The CP appears as a mound of tissue or as a bar just proximal to the esophageal introitus. Once the CP is visualized and exposed, the diverticuloscope is placed in suspension. If a nasogastric tube was used, it can be removed at this time. In order to obtain a sense of the size and depth of the CP, a right-angle probe can be used to palpate the CP mound.

Next, an incision is made through the CP mucosa. Different techniques have been described in the literature including electrocoagulation, CO_2 laser,[5,11,29–31] potassium titanyl phosphate laser,[25,32] harmonic scalpel,[33] and stapled approach for a diverticulectomy.[7,34,35] Endoscopic CPM originally used electrocoagulation to perform the myotomy, but shortly after the procedure was introduced, the laser technique was adopted. The laser technique was shown to be efficacious and safe with comparable outcomes to the electrocoagulation approach, but with less pain and shorter postoperative inability to eat.[25,36] The endoscopic stapling devices are not used in the absence of a diverticulum because the staplers cannot grasp the posterior aspect of the CP.[37]

CO_2 laser is now the tool of choice in the absence of a diverticulum given its ability to coagulate small vessels and minimize the spread of thermal damage, but utilization of the CO_2 laser is varied in the literature in regard to power and pulse used ranging from 3 to 12 W.[11,25,28,29] Pitman and Weissbrod[3] reports using the laser in a continuous-wave mode at a power of 6 W mechanically pulsed at 0.1 seconds on and 0.3 seconds off and graduating to use of a nonpulsed laser as experience is gained. Takes and colleagues[29] report use of 4W in continuous-wave motion, whereas Lawson and colleagues[10] use continuous wave type at 10 W power.

Once the mucosa is completely transected, there is a plane between the mucosa and muscle allowing the mucosa to be retracted for exposure of the whole height of the muscle. As the muscle is then incised with the laser in a midline vertical fashion, the muscle fibers should retract laterally. It is critical to transect all the muscle fibers in order to relieve the hypertonicity while being careful not to violate the buccopharyngeal fascia directly underneath. The buccopharyngeal fascia appears as a smooth, translucent white plane. In some patients, the buccopharyngeal fascia may be extremely thin or even nonexistent. When that is the case or if there is injury to the buccopharyngeal fascia, the areolar tissue of the retropharyngeal space is visible.[3] Care should be taken to keep the areolar tissue preserved to minimize risk of infection because pharyngeal contents will be contained by the areolar tissue if a leak occurs.[4]

The mucosa may heal by secondary intent or can be clipped,[27] sutured,[26,38] or fibrin glue applied.[11,29] When fibrin glue is applied, Pitman and Weissbrod[3] suggest placing an overlying suture in the mucosa to create a pocket in which the glue can sit and seal. The closure of the mucosa is thought to potentially reduce the incidence of postoperative cervical emphysema and mediastinitis risk while not compromising the functional outcome as it closes the access to the retropharyngeal space.[10,38] Huntley and colleagues[26] hypothesized that the closure of the mucosa also reduces postoperative discomfort and can hasten the advancement of the diet.

Technique: Endoscopic Management of Zenker's Diverticulum

Surgery, open or endoscopic, remains the definitive treatment for symptomatic ZD as well.

Surgical technique was initially focused on the diverticulum only before the role of the CP was understood in the pathogenesis of the ZD. Initially management of ZD was performed through an open technique with diverticulectomy, diverticulopexy, or diverticular inversion. Thereafter, the technique included myotomy of the common wall septum (CP) alone or in combination with treatment of the diverticulum depending on the size of the diverticulum (myotomy alone for <2 cm diverticula, suspension or resection if larger). As with the transcervical approach for isolated CPM, open diverticulectomy can have significant side effects, including recurrent laryngeal nerve injury, fistula formation, mediastinitis, and hematoma as well as risk for esophageal stricture and perforation.[39,40]

Rigid endoscopic approach: The endoscopic approach to ZD was first introduced in 1917, although not widely accepted at the time due to mediastinitis complications. Mosher described his method using a rigid endoscope to divide the common wall between the diverticulum and the esophagus. The method was modified almost a half century later with the use of the rigid endoscope and electrocautery to divide the septum in the 1960s and then further modification in 1990s using a CO_2 laser instead of electrocautery.[41,42] The use of endoscopic stapled devices to divide the CP bar was used in 1993 by Collard and colleagues[43] and became widely used.[44]

For the rigid endoscopic stapled technique, the patient is placed in supine position with neck hyperextension. Patients who have cervical disease precluding neck hyperextension are not candidates for the rigid endoscopic approach. The procedure is performed under general anesthesia. A bivalve diverticuloscope is placed with the anterior blade in the esophageal lumen and the posterior blade in the ZD. A telescope is passed and the septum is visualized with the scope placed in suspension. The endoscopic stapler is then introduced through the rigid endoscope with one blade of the stapler in the esophagus and the other in the diverticulum. Once fired, a diverticuloesophagostomy is created with the posterior wall of the esophagus stapled to the wall of the diverticulum and a common channel is created with the mucosal and muscular edges sealed by the staples.[40,43,45] In the stapled technique, a small remnant of septum usually remains due to the anvil of the stapler extending farther than the cutting apparatus. There are reports of sawing off the distal part of the anvil to eradicate the presence of the remnant septum, but this is problematic.[43] Because of this limitation and the need to divide 2 cm of CP, diverticula smaller than 3 cm are difficult to approach with this technique. In addition, limitations with jaw opening and neck extension lead to unsuccessful completion of the rigid endoscopy approach for nearly 30% of eligible patients.

Alternatives to the stapler in the rigid approach include the use of the harmonic scalpel with its use of ultrasonographic energy as a way to coagulate and seal the tissue before dividing it[33] and the use of the continuous wave of the CO_2 laser to create the division of the septum/CPM.[46] These alternatives still do not address limitations in access due to the factors mentioned earlier.

Flexible endoscopic approach: The flexible endoscopic approach to treating ZD is relatively novel with no standardization of approach. The procedure can be done under moderate sedation in an endoscopy suite or under general anesthesia in the operating room and is not limited by the need for neck hyperextension. As many of the patients with ZD are older adults who tend to be malnourished given their dysphagia, this has been shown to be a safe and effective method for treatment with the benefit of avoiding general anesthesia in these high-risk patients.

The flexible endoscopic approach with the use of monopolar forceps for cutting the ZD septum was introduced in 1995.[47,48] Alternatively, argon plasma coagulation (APC) can be used and has been shown to be safe and effective.[49] The optimal cutting technique is largely chosen based on preference of the endoscopist and his/her experience. However, unlike the rigid endoscopic approach, the CO_2 laser is not the safe choice for the flexible approach given positioning limitations.[40,50] The technique involves the same principle as the rigid endoscope technique: coagulation or cutting of the septum, and therefore the CP, between the esophagus and the diverticulum (**Fig. 5**). The size of the diverticulum dictates the safety of the procedure with one-stage approaches for small- to medium-sized ZD (up to 4 cm) and multiple stages in the approach for large ZD (>4 cm).[50]

As mentioned, the procedure can be performed under general anesthesia or conscious sedation after discussion with the anesthesiologist based on the patient's condition and comorbidities. Patients can be placed either supine or in the left lateral decubitus position. The technique of visualizing the septum is varied (see **Fig. 5A**). One option is utilization of a transparent hood or cap on the tip of the high-resolution video endoscope to help improve visualization and exposure as well as to stabilize the cautery instrument.[49,51] In addition, exposure can be aided by the placement of a nasogastric tube (NGT) as described in the isolated CPM approach. The NGT also acts as a protectant of the anterior wall of the esophagus from thermal injury during incision.[50] Alternatively, a soft diverticuloscope can be used to expose the septum acting like an overtube.[52,53] The special diverticuloscope for ZD will effectively straddle the septum, as in the rigid endoscopic technique, with a longer arm that will go into the esophagus and short arm into the diverticulum.[40,52]

Different techniques can be used to cut the tissue bridge between the ZD and the cervical esophagus, including APC probe, needle knife, harmonic scalpel, and bilateral forceps technique. In the APC probe technique, the incision is started 2 to 3 cm below the top of the tissue bridge. The endoscope is then pulled back caudally while applying APC. The treatment is stopped at least 1 cm above the bottom of the ZD to avoid perforation and the risk of mediastinitis. It is performed under high-power settings: APC 300 EEBE Generator at 99W and EEBE VIO-APC at 50W and "pulsed 1" APC mode[40,49] allowing a straight forward cutting direction without lateral spread of the beam.

The needle-knife technique is considered more advanced and harder to master.[40] Contrary to the APC technique, the needle-knife technique starts midline at the top of the septum (see **Fig. 5B**). Alternating between cut and coagulation mode, the septum is cut for at least two-thirds of its height to about 2 to 3 mm above the bottom of the diverticula.[54] An Endo Stitch can be placed in the septum at the start to put traction on the septum and pull it up toward the endoscope to provide better visualization and can be used in both the rigid and the flexible approach.[7,55] Once again, the incision must not extend past the inferior border of the diverticulum to prevent mediastinal perforation. A wide communicating channel is thus created between the ZD and the esophagus, and the outflow obstruction from the CP is relieved (see **Fig. 5C**). Some surgeons use only 1 or 2 endoclips at the base of the septal incision to prevent microperforation.[7,53,56,57] The authors prefer to close the entire mucosotomy transversely with clips (see **Fig. 5D**).

Other techniques include the bilateral forceps technique and the use of the harmonic scalpel. In the bilateral forceps technique, 2 endoclips are placed on each side of the cricopharyngeal bar and a needle-knife technique is used to dissect between the clips to the bottom of the diverticulum. It is thought that the 2 clips protect the septum sides.[40] With the harmonic scalpel technique, the soft diverticuloscope is inserted to allow for exposure. The harmonic scalpel is inserted with the shears open. They are then closed around the septum with the machine set to minimum value of

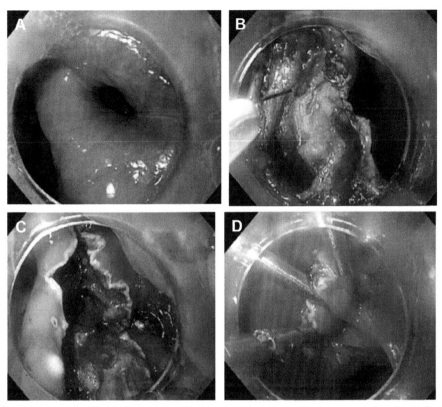

Fig. 5. Technique of the flexible endoscopic treatment of a ZD. (*A*) Diverticulum is visualized and the CP septum dividing the ZD from the esophageal inlet is seen in the center of the screen. (*B*) Myotomy of the CP septum being performed. The muscle fibers are retracting laterally as cut. (*C*) Completed mucosotomy and myotomy. (*D*) Closure of the mucosotomy with clips.

3 and maximum of 5. The scalpel is then activated, and it seals and divides the septum.[33] However, neck extension may limit the use of this rigid instrument. Submucosal dissection knives such as the Dual-Knife (Olympus endotherapy, Tokyo, Japan) and HybridKnife (Erbe, Tubingen, Germany) are also used to perform the myotomy.

Postoperative Care

A wide variety of postoperative protocols exist without any convincing studies to support a standardized approach regarding timing of swallow studies, duration of antibiotics, and advancement of diet. The placement of NGT postoperatively is avoided given the potential for creating a false passage and its proximity to the incision.[10] Positive pressure ventilation should also be avoided when possible, especially in patients who had injury to their buccopharyngeal fascia or thin fascia to decrease the incidence of cervical emphysema.[3] Patients are placed on antibiotics prophylactically at the start of the surgery and continued for up to 7 days postoperatively but typically for 2 postoperative doses. Thin barium swallow studies

are performed as early as the morning of postoperative day one or later at postoperative day 3 with the advancement to a clear liquid diet if there is no evidence of leak. Our standard approach is for NPO status on the day of the procedure, followed by a contrast swallow the following morning to rule out leak and assure adequacy of myotomy and mucosal closure, followed by advancement to liquid diet. A liquid diet is continued for 7 to 10 days to avoid disrupting the healing mucosotomy. If a leak is detected on swallow study, the patient may be returned to the operating room for attempted sealing with clips and/or endoscopic gluing. Leaks are uncommon in the authors' experience.

Clinical Results in the Literature

Studies that report on isolated endoscopic CPM without ZD are limited and have small sample sizes with a mixed cause of underlying CP dysfunction resulting in multiple confounding factors when examining the literature. However, in the multiple small case series performed examining institutions' experience with endoscopic CPM, favorable outcomes have been reported with minimal complications. Examples include Dale and colleagues[27] who described 38 patients at their institution with a statistically significant improvement in swallowing and reflux scores and a 2.6% complication rate with 1 patient developing mediastinitis (the only reported case in the literature) and 4 with recurrent dysphagia. In their series, Takes and colleagues[29] described 10 patients without a ZD who underwent an endoscopic CPM. Most patients had improvement in symptoms, except one patient with reported recurrent dysphagia. There were no complications reported. Lawson and colleagues[11] reported no complications in their 29 patient series. In a systemic review of CPM in neurologic disease, there was insufficient evidence to support the effectiveness of the CPM in relief or recurrence of symptoms.[58]

Comparing open to the endoscopic approach, Dauer and colleagues[28] described 14 patients who underwent endoscopic approach to 8 who underwent the open technique. They revealed a similar success rate between the 2 approaches; however, the endoscopic approach was associated with shorter operative times and hospital stays. The complication rate was also similar in the 2 groups, but the open approach had more major complications, including a pharyngocutaneous fistula. More recently, Huntley and colleagues[26] compared patients with cricopharyngeal hyperfunction who underwent an open approach (38 cases) with those who underwent endoscopic approach (41 cases). They found a significant improvement in surgical time and symptomatic outcome in the endoscopic group, but no difference in complication rate, time to oral intake, or length of hospital stay.

In treatment of ZD, there exists much heterogeneity in the literature. In addition to differences in overall techniques (open, rigid endoscopic, or flexible endoscopic) there is also much variation within these subsets on how the procedures are performed and there are no randomized trials to study the differences between the overall techniques. Overall the endoscopic technique, both rigid and flexible, has been shown to have advantages over open surgery, including shorter operating time, less morbidity, shorter length of stay, and quicker time to oral intake postoperatively.[40,59] In a larger series, Chang and colleagues[60] compared open and endoscopic approaches with a higher complication rate reported in open (11.8%) versus endoscopic (5.5%), a longer hospital stay in open (7.6 vs 1.8 days), and 4.5 days until diets were resumed in open with only 1 day in the endoscopic approach.

In a recent study on the evolving management of ZD, Jones and colleagues[7] retrospectively reviewed 62 patients who underwent either open (39 patients) or endoscopic (23 patients) technique. Of the endoscopically treated patients, 8 had a rigid approach and 15 had a flexible approach. The endoscopic myotomy was attempted in 35 patients, but completed endoscopically only in 23. Reasons for converting to open in the rigid approach included inability to properly position the diverticuloscope for visualization, whereas in the flexible approach, a small diverticulum was the sole reason for converting to open. The rigid and endoscopic techniques were equally effective in relieving symptoms of dysphagia. Postoperative complications in open, rigid, and flexible approaches were 13%, 25%, and 7%, respectively, with a trend toward decreased major complications in the flexible approach (1 open and 1 rigid esophageal perforation). Length of stay was lower in the flexible approach.

Twenty studies including a total of 813 patients were examined in a recent systemic review and meta-analysis of flexible endoscopic treatment for ZD. There was a reported pooled success rate of 91% with an adverse events rate of 11.3% and an 11% recurrence rate.[61] The potentially life-threatening complications encountered including bleeding and perforation were managed conservatively in all but 2 patients in whom drainage of an abscess was necessary. This analysis demonstrated that a flexible endoscopic approach is safe and effective, with rates of success and adverse events comparable to open and rigid approach, but with the added benefit of no neck mobilization limitations and the ability to do the procedure without general anesthesia. It also demonstrated a large degree of heterogeneity in the flexible endoscopic approach with no current standardization in the procedure itself or the postoperative care.

In a review of 89 patients, the prognostic variables that determined clinical success in the flexible approach were assessed. It was further validated that the flexible approach is a safe and effective approach and found that treatment success correlates with the length of the septotomy and the size of the ZD. Variables for failure at 6 months were a septotomy length less than 2.5 cm and a pretreatment ZD greater than 5 cm.[62] Additional literature has shown that presence of a small diverticulum makes the procedure more difficult and that open techniques can possibly provide better symptom relief for small diverticula given the short size of the septum to cut.[7,39] This limitation may perhaps be overcome by tunneling the myotomy for at least 2 cm and completely closing the mucosa with clips.

In general, endoscopic CPM with or without ZD offers shorter operative time, less morbidity, and improved cosmesis with a scar-free surgery compared with the open technique. Current literature suggests that the rate of both minor and major complications can be compared favorably with the open approach. There is a need for further large, prospective studies to compare the different approaches and to aid in the standardization of the novel technique in the flexible endoscopic approach.

Summary

Endoscopic CPM has been demonstrated to be a safe and efficacious procedure with favorable outcomes for the treatment of cricopharyngeal dysfunction with or without ZD. It is a less invasive approach with decreased morbidity compared with the open approach and minimal reported complications. This novel technique has continued to gain popularity since its introduction in the 1990s. A thorough workup of patients to make the diagnosis of isolated cricopharyngeal dysfunction with or without ZD is necessary for the proper selection of patients. Continued studies on a larger scale are needed to further refine the techniques and explore the outcomes and complications of patients undergoing endoscopic CPM and developing standardization for the procedure.

ENDOSCOPIC PYLOROMYOTOMY
Introduction

Gastroparesis is a chronic, functional disorder characterized by symptoms of delayed gastric emptying including nausea and vomiting. In gastroparesis, quality of life can significantly suffer.[63] The development of gastroparesis may stem from several causes. First-line therapies for the disease process usually include medication and diet modification, but as the disease progresses and becomes refractory to medications, many patients need endoscopic or surgical options to address their gastroparesis. These interventional options include a spectrum of treatments including injection of botulinum toxin into the pylorus, endoscopic transpyloric stent placement, gastric electrical stimulation devices, laparoscopic or open pyloroplasty, and even gastric bypass or gastrectomy in advanced cases.[64] In 2013, the first reports of the performance of endoscopic pyloromyotomy in humans was published by Khashab and colleagues,[65] building on the principles from the peroral endoscopic myotomy technique for achalasia. Since its recent introduction, several

other centers have detailed their technique of this novel approach to treating gastroparesis. The authors aim to describe the peroral pyloromyotomy (POP) indications as well as technique.

Indications and Diagnosis

Gastric emptying is a highly coordinated effort of impulses between different regions of the stomach and duodenum with extrinsic modulation by the central nervous system. These impulses work together to deliver food distally in the gastrointestinal (GI) tract. The major events that lead to normal gastric emptying include fundic relaxation, antral contractions, and pyloric relaxation to allow food to exit the stomach. The pathophysiology of gastroparesis includes 2 major components: the alteration of gastric motility causing atony of the stomach and an increase in pyloric tone.[66] Many of the treatment options, including POP, target the pylorus to increase the ease of the passage of the food bolus distally into the duodenum.[63,64]

The development of gastroparesis is multifactorial, and the potential causes of the disease include diabetes, medication-induced (particularly narcotics), postsurgical/vagus nerve injury, gastroesophageal reflux disease, hypertrophic pyloric stenosis, neurologic disorders, collagen vascular disorders, or idiopathic causes. Gastroparesis can present with a wide range of symptoms such as early satiety, nausea, vomiting, upper abdominal discomfort, and bloating. As the symptoms are broad and mimic many other diseases, a thorough workup to diagnose gastroparesis is necessary.

Gastroparesis is a diagnosis of exclusion by demonstrating that other potential reversible causes of symptoms are not causing the delayed gastric emptying. The diagnosis is made on a clinical suspicion, and functional studies of the GI tract are used to confirm the suspicion. The evaluation of the patients suspected to have delayed gastric emptying can be thought of in a stepwise approach.[63] In the initial investigation, a thorough history and physical examination are of key importance. In addition, blood tests including CBC and CMP should be sent. Then an evaluation of organic disorders should occur. This phase includes an upper endoscopy to evaluate for any mechanical obstruction or mucosal lesions such as tumor or stricture. Barium upper GI series with small bowel follow-through can also be used to identify any mechanical obstruction. The gold standard test is a solid-phase gastric emptying study to confirm delayed gastric emptying.[63,67,68] A wireless motility catheter can also be used and is helpful to differentiate patients with isolated gastroparesis from those patients with global gut dysfunction.[67]

Once gastroparesis is diagnosed, patients are usually followed by a multidisciplinary team, including gastroenterologists, surgeons, nutritionists, psychologists, and pain management experts.[67] Initial treatment is often with dietary modifications and medications, including prokinetics, antiemetics, and analgesics, but there is a varied, unpredictable response to these treatments and often further therapy is indicated.[64] Endoscopic intrapyloric botulinum toxin injections are a commonly used therapy, as well as a diagnostic modality to predict response to pyloric division. Low-dose injection in the pylorus muscle decreases contractility and at higher doses, directly affects muscle tone.[69] The effect of the botulinum toxin injection is temporary, only lasting approximately 1 to 5 months,[70] and there have even been 2 controlled trials that found no difference between botulinum toxin injection and a saline solution injection.[71,72] Much like the CPM, response to the botulinum toxin injection can predict a good response to a pyloromyotomy. The endoscopic pyloromyotomy has become an appealing minimally invasive therapeutic option for patients with refractory symptoms given that the distention and disruption of the pylorus can result in symptomatic improvement[65] and because it is less invasive than more aggressive surgical approaches.

Technique

All reports of the POP procedure were performed in the operating room under general anesthesia. Given that the patients have poor gastric emptying, it is important that in preparation for the surgery, patients are placed on a full liquid diet for 2 days followed by a day of a clear liquid diet before the procedure to reduce the risk of aspiration.[67] The patient is placed in a supine position and intubated after the induction of anesthesia. A cap is placed on the standard gastroscope with a 2.8-mm working channel and the cap is secured with tape. The cap can aid in retracting the mucosa when in the intramural tunnel. CO_2 gas is used for insufflation throughout the procedure. The electrosurgical unit settings are applied, with reports of the Erbe VIO 300D unit being used with the cut mode at 50W on Effect 3 and coagulation set to Spray-Coag Effect 2 at 50W.[65,67]

A diagnostic endoscopy is performed to start, and all remaining food or debris is removed for adequate visualization of the pylorus. A mix of saline, methylene blue, and epinephrine is injected approximately 3 to 5 cm proximal to the pylorus. There are conflicting reports of placing the injection on either the lesser curve or the greater curve.[65,67,73] Earlier literature reports injecting on the greater curve, but more recent technique has found that placing the injection in the lesser curve leads to the need for a shorter tunnel and more closely approximates the tissue.[67,73]

Next, an approximately 1.5 cm transverse incision is made into the mucosa where the injection was placed using the triangle tip knife or Hydro-Knife on cut energy. Once the incision is made, the posterior lip of the mucosa can be retracted downward to allow for the cap and endoscope to be introduced into the submucosa. Now, with the knife on coagulation, a submucosal tunnel is created and extended just beyond the white pyloric muscle to approximately 0.5 cm into the duodenal bulb.[65]

The pylorus muscle is now exposed and the muscle fibers can be divided with the knife again on coagulation setting. With the aid of pressure from the cap, the myotomy starts distally and comes back proximally one layer at a time until completely divided through the inner circular and oblique muscle bundles while preserving the outer longitudinal muscle layer. Care must be taken at the distal edge of the pylorus because the duodenal mucosa drapes over in a perpendicular fashion therefore increasing the risk of inadvertent perforation.[74] There have been reports of placing an endoclip in the pyloric channel and using fluoroscopic guidance to identify the pyloric ring.[75,76] There is little data to guide the length of myotomy. In a study using an ex vivo porcine stomach model, different myotomy lengths (1, 2, 3, or 4 cm) were compared, and it was determined that a 3-cm pyloromyotomy was best for the large animals and 2 cm for a small stomach series.[77] After completion and verification of hemostasis, the endoscope can be withdrawn from the tunnel. The mucosotomy is closed with endoscopic clips. Patients are extubated at the end of the procedure.

Postoperative Care

Patients are kept NPO initially postoperatively until an upper GI contrast study with water-soluble contrast can be performed the following morning. If the study is normal, with no signs of a leak, then a clear liquid diet is started. Patients are typically discharged on postoperative day 1 on a clear liquid diet and advance at home to a full liquid diet for approximately 7 to 10 days. Patients are given a dose of antibiotics preoperatively, and the antibiotics are continued for 2 doses postoperatively for prophylaxis. A proton pump inhibitor and sucralfate therapy for 6 weeks postoperatively are used to prevent ulceration at the mucosotomy site.[67]

Clinical Results in the Literature

Given its relatively recent introduction to practice, there are limited studies on POP especially in comparing it to a laparoscopic pyloromyotomy and other endoscopic treatment modalities for gastroparesis and examining long-term results. Overall, the POP has been shown to be safe with limited complications.[66,67,73,74,76] In their paper describing their technique for POP, Allemang and colleagues[67] completed 57 POPs at their institution with no leaks, obstructions, or other complications reported in their short-term follow-up. The procedure on average took 41 minutes, and there was an overall improvement of symptoms as measured by the validated Gastroparesis Cardinal System Index.

Shlomovitz and colleagues[74] performed POP in 7 female patients with technical success in all cases. Six of the seven patients experienced significant symptomatic improvements. One patient did not respond to POP and went on to require a laparoscopic pyloromyotomy, which of note also failed to improve symptoms. Of 5 patients who had short-term follow-up gastric emptying studies, normal gastric emptying was reported in 4 (80%) of the patients. Postoperative complications included hospital-acquired pneumonia and an upper GI bleed 2 weeks postoperatively from a pyloric channel ulcer requiring transfusion and reclipping. In another article, Dacha and colleagues[76] described their outcomes and quality of life assessment after POP in 13 patients. They reported a mean operative time of 49 minutes and a mean length of hospital stay of 2.5 days. They had no adverse events occur, and using the SF36 questionnaire, a significant improvement in quality of life was sustained through the 6-month follow-up. The mean myotomy length was approximately 3 cm in their reports.

The small number of studies with just short-term follow-up limits the ability to demonstrate the full impact of POP on the care of patients with gastroparesis, but these early studies do suggest that it is a safe and effective treatment modality with low rate of complications and high rate of improvement in symptoms. Continued studies and more data with longer-term follow-up are needed in this novel technique.

SUMMARY

Gastroparesis is a difficult chronic disease with many treatment options all with varied results for individual patients. There is no gold standard in the treatment of this disease. Peroral endoscopic pyloromyotomy is a new technique that has shown promising results in terms of its safety, complication profile, and symptom improvement in a minimally invasive approach that is appealing to many patients. As further data emerge on the technique, long-term efficacy of the procedure will be better understood and compared with other techniques in the treatment of gastroparesis.

REFERENCES

1. Haapaniemi JJ, Laurikainen EA, Pulkkinen J, et al. Botulinum toxin in the treatment of cricopharyngeal dysphagia. Dysphagia 2001;16(3):171–5.
2. Tieu BH, Hunter JG. Management of cricopharyngeal dysphagia with and without zenker's diverticulum. Thorac Surg Clin 2011;21(4):511–7.
3. Pitman M, Weissbrod P. Endoscopic cricopharyngeal myotomy. Oper Tech Otolaryngol - Head Neck Surg 2011;22:135–41.
4. Chang CWD, Liou SS, Netterville JL. Anatomic study of laser-assisted endoscopic cricopharyngeus myotomy. Ann Otol Rhinol Laryngol 2005;114(12):897–901.
5. Pitman M, Weissbrod P. Endoscopic CO_2 laser cricopharyngeal myotomy. Laryngoscope 2009;119(1):45–53.
6. Zaninotto G, Costantini M, Boccù C, et al. Functional and morphological study of the cricopharyngeal muscle in patients with Zenker's diverticulum. Br J Surg 1996;83(9):1263–7.
7. Jones D, Aloraini A, Gowing S, et al. Evolving management of Zenker's diverticulum in the endoscopic era: a north american experience. World J Surg 2016;40(6):1390–6.
8. Cook IJ, Blumbergs P, Cash K, et al. Structural abnormalities of the cricopharyngeus muscle in patients with pharyngeal (Zenker's) diverticulum. J Gastroenterol Hepatol 1992;7(6):556–62.
9. Bammer T, Salassa JR, Klingler PJ. Comparison of methods for determining cricopharyngeal intrabolus pressure in normal patients as possible indicator for cricopharyngeal myotomy. Otolaryngol Neck Surg 2002;127(4):299–308.
10. Lawson G, Remacle M. Endoscopic cricopharyngeal myotomy: indications and technique. Curr Opin Otolaryngol Head Neck Surg 2006;14:437–41.
11. Lawson G, Remacle M, Jamart J, et al. Endoscopic CO2 laser-assisted surgery for cricopharyngeal dysfunction. Eur Arch Otorhinolaryngol 2003;260(9):475–80.
12. Solt J, Bajor J, Moizs M, et al. Primary cricopharyngeal dysfunction: treatment with balloon catheter dilatation. Gastrointest Endosc 2001;54(6):767–71.

13. Zepeda-Gómez S, Loza AM, Valdovinos F, et al. Case report: endoscopic balloon catheter dilation for treatment of primary cricopharyngeal dysfunction. Dig Dis Sci 2004;49(10):1612–4.

14. Ahsan SF, Meleca RJ, Dworkin James P. Botulinum toxin injection of the cricopharyngeus muscle for the treatment of dysphagia. Otolaryngol Neck Surg 2000;122(5):691–5.

15. Kim M-S, Kim G-W, Rho Y-S, et al. Office-based electromyography-guided botulinum toxin injection to the cricopharyngeus muscle: optimal patient selection and technique. Ann Otol Rhinol Laryngol 2017;126(5):349–56.

16. Murry T, Wasserman T, Carrau RL, et al. Injection of botulinum toxin A for the treatment of dysfunction of the upper esophageal sphincter. Am J Otolaryngol 2005;26(3):157–62.

17. Kelly EA, Koszewski IJ, Jaradeh SS, et al. Botulinum toxin injection for the treatment of upper esophageal sphincter dysfunction. Ann Otol Rhinol Laryngol 2013;122(2):100–8.

18. Blitzer A, Brin MF. Use of botulinum toxin for diagnosis and management of cricopharyngeal achalasia. Otolaryngol Neck Surg 1997;116(3):328–30.

19. Cook IJ. Oropharyngeal dysphagia. Gastroenterol Clin North Am 2009;38(3):411–31.

20. Schneider I, Pototschnig C, Thumfart WF, et al. Treatment of dysfunction of the cricopharyngeal muscle with botulinum a toxin: introduction of a new, noninvasive method. Ann Otol Rhinol Laryngol 1994;103(1):31–5.

21. Kocdor P, Siegel ER, Tulunay-Ugur OE. Cricopharyngeal dysfunction: a systematic review comparing outcomes of dilatation, botulinum toxin injection, and myotomy. Laryngoscope 2016;126(1):135–41.

22. Marston AP, Maldonado FJ, Ravi K, et al. Treatment of oropharyngeal dysphagia secondary to idiopathic cricopharyngeal bar: surgical cricopharyngeal muscle myotomy versus dilation. Am J Otolaryngol 2016; 37(6):507–12.

23. Brigand C, Ferraro P, Martin J, et al. Risk factors in patients undergoing cricopharyngeal myotomy. Br J Surg 2007;94(8):978–83.

24. Ross ER, Green R, Auslander MO, et al. Cricopharyngeal myotomy: management of cervical dysphagia. Otolaryngol Neck Surg 1982;90(4): 434–41.

25. Halvorson DJ, Kuhn FA. Transmucosal cricopharyngeal myotomy with the potassium-titanyl-phosphate laser in the treatment of cricopharyngeal dysmotility. Ann Otol Rhinol Laryngol 1994;103(3): 173–7.

26. Huntley C, Boon M, Spiegel J. Open vs. endoscopic cricopharyngeal myotomy; Is there a difference? Am J Otolaryngol 2017;38(4):405–7.

27. Dale OT, Mackeith S, Burgess CA, et al. Functional outcomes following endoscopic laser cricopharyngeal myotomy with mucosal repair. Eur Arch Oto-rhino-laryngology 2014;271(6): 1631–4.

28. Dauer E, Salassa J, Iuga L, et al. Endoscopic laser vs open approach for cricopharyngeal myotomy. Otolaryngol Neck Surg 2006;134(5):830–5.

29. Takes RP, Van Den Hoogen FJA, Marres HAM. Endoscopic myotomy of the cricopharyngeal muscle with CO_2 laser surgery. Head Neck 2005; 27(8):703–9.

30. Bergeron JL, Chhetri DK. Indications and outcomes of endoscopic CO_2 laser cricopharyngeal myotomy. Laryngoscope 2014;124(4):950–4.

31. Guideline National Institute for Health and Care Excellence (NICE). Endoscopic carbon dioxide laser cricopharyngeal myotomy for relief of oropharyngeal dysphagia. 2016. p. 1–7.

32. Kuhn FA, Bent JP. Zenker's diverticulotomy using the KTP/532 laser. Laryngoscope 1992;102(8): 946–50.

33. Fama AF, Moore EJ, Kasperbauer JL. Harmonic scalpel in the treatment of Zenker's diverticulum. Laryngoscope 2009;119(7):1265–9.

34. Bizzotto A, Iacopini F, Landi R, et al. Zenker's diverticulum: exploring treatment options. Acta Otorhinolaryngol Ital 2013;33:219–29.

35. Pescarus R, Shlomovitz E, Sharata AM, et al. Transoral cricomyotomy using a flexible endoscope: technique and clinical outcomes. Surg Endosc 2016; 30(5):1784–9.

36. McKenna JA, Dedo HH. Cricopharyngeal myotomy: indications and technique. Ann Otol Rhinol Laryngol 1992;101(3):216–21.

37. Ashman A, Dale OT, Baldwin DL. Management of isolated cricopharyngeal dysfunction: systematic review. J Laryngol Otol 2016;130(7):611–5.

38. Ho AS, Morzaria S, Damrose EJ. Carbon dioxide laser—assisted endoscopic cricopharyngeal myotomy with primary mucosal closure. Ann Otol Rhinol Laryngol 2011;120(1):33–9.

39. Gutschow CA, Hamoir M, Rombaux P, et al. Management of pharyngoesophageal (Zenker's) diverticulum: which technique? Ann Thorac Surg 2002; 74(5):1677–83.

40. Dzeletovic I, Ekbom DC, Baron TH. Flexible endoscopic and surgical management of Zenker's diverticulum. Expert Rev Gastoenterol Hepatol 2012;6(4): 449–66.

41. Lippert BM, Folz BJ, Rudert HH, et al. Management of Zenker's diverticulum and postlaryngectomy pseudodiverticulum with the CO_2 laser. Otolaryngol Neck Surg 1999;121(6):809–14.

42. Zbären P, Schär P, Tschopp L, et al. Surgical treatment of zenker's diverticulum: transcutaneous diverticulectomy versus microendoscopic myotomy of the cricopharyngeal muscle with CO_2 laser. Otolaryngol Neck Surg 1999;121(4):482–7.

43. Collard JM, Otte JB, Kestens PJ. Endoscopic stapling technique of esophagodiverticulostomy for Zenker's diverticulum. Ann Thorac Surg 1993; 56(3):573–6.

44. Scher RL, Richtsmeier WJ. Endoscopic staple-assisted esophagodiverticulostomy for zenker's diverticulum. Laryngoscope 1996;106:951–6.

45. Richtsmeier WJ. Endoscopic management of Zenker diverticulum: the staple-assisted approach. Am J Med 2003;115(3 SUPPL. 1):1–4.

46. Visser LJ, Hardillo JAU, Monserez DA, et al. Zenker's diverticulum: rotterdam experience. Eur Arch Otorhino-laryngology 2016;273(9):2755–63.

47. Ischioka S, Sakai F, Maluf Filho J, et al. Endoscopic incision of zenker's diverticula. Endocrine 1995;6: 433–7.

48. Mulder CJ, den Hartog G, Robijn RJ, et al. Flexible endoscopic treatment of zenker's diverticulum: a new approach. Endoscopy 1995;6:438–42.

49. Rabenstein T, May A, Michel J, et al. Argon plasma coagulation for flexible endoscopic Zenker's diverticulotomy. Endoscopy 2006;39(2):233–45.

50. Mulder CJ, Costamagna G, Sakai P. Zenker's diverticulum: treatment using a flexible endoscope. Endoscopy 2001;33(11):991–7.

51. Christiaens P, De Roock W, Van Olmen A, et al. Treatment of Zenker's diverticulum through a flexible endoscope with a transparent oblique-end hood attached to the tip and a monopolar forceps. Endoscopy 2006;39(2):137–40.

52. Evrard S, Le Moine O, Hassid S, et al. Zenker's diverticulum: a new endoscopic treatment with a soft diverticuloscope. Gastrointest Endosc 2003;58(1): 116–20.

53. Costamagna G, Iancopini F, Tringali A, et al. Flexible endoscopic Zenker's diverticulotomy: cap-assisted technique vs. diverticuloscope-assisted technique. Endoscopy 2007;39(2):146–52.

54. Vogelsang A, Preiss C, Neuhaus H, et al. Endotherapy of Zenker's diverticulum using the needle-knife technique: long-term follow up. Endoscopy 2006; 39(2):131–6.

55. Bonavina L, Nosadini A, Bardini R, et al. Primary treatment of esophageal achalasia long-term results of myotomy and dor fundoplication. Surg Endosc Other Interv Tech 2012;26(10): 2856–61.

56. Manno M, Manta R, Caruso A, et al. Alternative endoscopic treatment of Zenker's diverticulum: a case series (with video). Gastrointest Endosc 2014;79(1):168–70.

57. Laquière A, Grandval P, Arpurt JP, et al. Interest of submucosal dissection knife for endoscopic treatment of Zenker's diverticulum. Surg Endosc Other Interv Tech 2015;29(9):2802–10.

58. Gilheaney Ó, Kerr P, Béchet S, et al. Effectiveness of endoscopic cricopharyngeal myotomy in adults with neurological disease: systematic review. J Laryngol Otol 2016;130(12):1077–85.

59. De-La-Morena-Madrigal EJ, Perez-Arellano E, Rodriguez-Garcia I. Flexible endoscopic treatment of Zenker's diverticulum: thirteen years' experience in Spain. Rev Esp Enferm Dig 2016; 108(6):297–303.

60. Chang CY, Payyapilli RJ, Scher RL. Endoscopic staple diverticulostomy for zenker's diverticulum: review of literature and experience in 159 consecutive cases. Laryngoscope 2003;113(6):957–65.

61. Ishaq S, Hassan C, Antonello A, et al. Flexible endoscopic treatment for Zenker's diverticulum: a systematic review and meta-analysis. Gastrointest Endosc 2016;83(6):1076–89.

62. Costamagna G, Iacopini F, Bizzotto A, et al. Prognostic variables for the clinical success of flexible endoscopic septotomy of Zenker's diverticulum. Gastrointest Endosc 2016;83(4):765–73.

63. Parkman HP, Hasler WL, Fisher RS. American gastroenterological association technical review on the diagnosis and treatment of gastroparesis. Gastroenterology 2004;127(5):1592–622.

64. McCarty TR, Rustagi T. Endoscopic treatment of gastroparesis. World J Gastroenterol 2015;21(22): 6842–9.

65. Khashab MA, Stein E, Clarke JO, et al. Gastric peroral endoscopic myotomy for refractory gastroparesis: first human endoscopic pyloromyotomy (with video). Gastrointest Endosc 2013;78(5):764–8.

66. Gonzalez JM, Lestelle V, Benezech A, et al. Gastric per-oral endoscopic myotomy with antropyloromyotomy in the treatment of refractory gastroparesis: clinical experience with follow-up and scintigraphic evaluation (with video). Gastrointest Endosc 2017; 85(1):132–9.

67. Allemang MT, Strong AT, Haskins IN, et al. How I do it: Per-Oral Pyloromyotomy (POP). J Gastrointest Surg 2017;21(11):1963–8.

68. Camilleri M, Parkman HP, Shafi MA, et al. Clinical guideline: management of gastroparesis. Am J Gastroenterol 2013;108(1):18–37.

69. James AN, Ryan JP, Parkman HP. Inhibitory effects of botulinum toxin on pyloric and antral smooth muscle. Am J Physiol Gastrointest Liver Physiol 2003; 285(2):G291–7.

70. Bromer MQ, Friedenberg F, Miller LS, et al. Endoscopic pyloric injection of botulinum toxin A for the treatment of refractory gastroparesis. Gastrointest Endosc 2005;61(7):833–9.

71. Friedenberg FK, Palit A, Parkman HP, et al. Botulinum toxin A for the treatment of delayed gastric emptying. Am J Gastroenterol 2008;103(2):416–23.

72. Arts J, Holvoet L, Caenepeel P, et al. Clinical trial: a randomized-controlled crossover study of intrapyloric injection of botulinum toxin in gastroparesis. Aliment Pharmacol Ther 2007;26(9):1251–8.

73. Rodriguez JH, Haskins IN, Strong AT, et al. Per oral endoscopic pyloromyotomy for refractory gastroparesis: initial results from a single institution. Surg Endosc Other Interv Tech 2017;31(12):1–8.

74. Shlomovitz E, Pescarus R, Cassera MA, et al. Early human experience with per-oral endoscopic pyloromyotomy (POP). Surg Endosc 2015;29(3): 543–51.

75. Xue HB, Fan HZ, Meng XM, et al. Fluoroscopy-guided gastric peroral endoscopic pyloromyotomy (G-POEM): a more reliable and efficient method for treatment of refractory gastroparesis. Surg Endosc Other Interv Tech 2017;31(11):4617–24.

76. Dacha S, Mekaroonkamol P, Li L, et al. Outcomes and quality-of-life assessment after gastric per-oral endoscopic pyloromyotomy (with video). Gastrointest Endosc 2017;86(2):282–9.

77. Jung Y, Lee J, Gromski MA, et al. Assessment of the length of myotomy in peroral endoscopic pyloromyotomy (G-POEM) using a submucosal tunnel technique (video). Surg Endosc Other Interv Tech 2015;29(8):2377–84.

Extraluminal Approaches to Gastroesophageal Reflux Disease

James M. Tatum, MD[a], John C. Lipham, MD[b,c],*

KEYWORDS

- GERD • LINX • Magnetic sphincter augmentation • Fundoplication • EndoStim

KEY POINTS

- Before considering surgical therapy of gastroesophageal reflux disease, it is incumbent on the surgeon to confirm the presence of pathologic reflux, adequate esophageal motility, and the absence of other explanatory or complicating esophageal or gastric diseases.
- The gold standard extraluminal surgical intervention for gastroesophageal reflux disease is complete or partial gastric fundoplication of the esophagus and hiatal hernia repair.
- Novel modalities, including the LINX and EndoStim, offer less invasive and perhaps equivocal or even superior alternatives to fundoplication in appropriately selected patients.

INTRODUCTION

The surgical treatment of gastroesophageal reflux disease (GERD) has been one of the great successes of laparoscopy in the past decades, even in the face of major advances in the medical therapy of the condition. The obesity epidemic and modern behavioral vices make reflux a disease of relatively high prevalence (between 3% and 33%), which coupled with growing concerns of the side effects of popular proton pump inhibitors used to treat the symptoms of the disease make surgical intervention both attractive to and indicated for patients with GERD.[1]

The surgical therapies available to treat GERD have evolved and multiplied over the past decades. The gastric fundoplication, once performed through a thoracic or open transabdominal approach has become in all but the most complicated cases a transabdominal procedure, and now a nearly universally laparoscopic procedure. Options for fundoplication include the complete or partial fundoplication as well as the maturing extraluminal magnetic sphincter augmentation device and the experimental lower esophageal sphincter (LES) stimulation device. In addition to a host of procedures to address the tone of the LES, understanding the importance of the hiatus in the physiology of antireflux surgery is of tantamount importance.[2,3]

DIAGNOSTIC STUDIES

GERD typically presents with well-known symptoms of water-brash, regurgitation, and pyrosis or dysphagia. Atypical symptoms and complaints are also common, including vomiting, chronic cough or laryngitis, and even serious lung or sinus diseases. Some combination of these symptoms is sensitive but not specific for reflux disease.

Disclosure: Dr J.M. Tatum has nothing to disclose. J.C. Lipham is a paid consultant for Johnson & Johnson Corporation.

[a] Department of Surgery, Division of General and Laparoscopic Surgery, Keck School of Medicine, University of Southern California, 1450 San Pablo Street HCC 4, Suite 6200, Los Angeles, CA 90033, USA; [b] Division of General Surgery, Keck School of Medicine, University of Southern California, 1450 San Pablo Street HCC 4, Suite 6200, Los Angeles, CA 90033, USA; [c] Division of Minimally Invasive Surgery, Keck School of Medicine, University of Southern California, 1450 San Pablo Street HCC 4, Suite 6200, Los Angeles, CA 90033, USA
* Corresponding author. 1450 San Pablo Street HCC 4, Suite 6200, Los Angeles, CA 90033.
E-mail address: John.Lipham@med.usc.edu

Thorac Surg Clin 28 (2018) 521–526
https://doi.org/10.1016/j.thorsurg.2018.07.003
1547-4127/18/© 2018 Elsevier Inc. All rights reserved.

The diagnosis of reflux disease requires several key diagnostic studies. We routinely use 4 diagnostic studies. An upper endoscopy (EGD) is key to rule out malignant or anatomic defects of the esophagus or stomach as well as to visualize the distal esophagus and facilitates biopsy of potentially metaplastic or dysplastic tissue. While conducting the EGD, the second test, a pH study is facilitated when a detachable 48-hour to 96-hour pH probe is left on the esophageal wall providing a measurement of esophageal acid exposure. We primarily use the video esophagogram (VEG) to assess motility of the esophagus and as the most sensitive study to diagnose and assess the size of hiatal hernia, particularly those that are small.[4] The fourth routine study is esophageal manometry to formally characterize esophageal motility. Rarely, a symptomatic patient will have symptoms consistent with reflux or other esophageal dysmotility disorder, which results in equivocal or negative DeMeester score, in which case we pursue impedance studies, particularly in cases in which we suspect alkaline reflux. In patients with questionable motility on VEG or manometry, we advocate partial fundoplication. Patients with nausea and vomiting as the predominant symptoms merit a nuclear medicine gastric emptying study to assess for gastroparesis. Failure to adequately diagnose poor gastric emptying or an occult esophageal motility disorder can result in disastrous outcomes for the patient and surgeon.

In patients with a DeMeester score of greater than 14.72, anatomically normal EGD without cancer, and a VEG with adequate motility, we offer a complete fundoplication or magnetic sphincter augmentation. In patients with impaired motility we offer a partial fundoplication, preferentially the posterior 270° wrap. As discussed later, in the most complex patients we consider a Roux-en-Y procedure.

FUNDOPLICATION

GERD is a result of an incompetent LES that results in transient or basal low LES tone.[5] This incompetence is primarily the result of a weak lower esophageal smooth muscle tone, and is contributed to by a laxity of the diaphragmatic crural or a hiatal hernia.[2,3] The object of the fundoplication, regardless of approach or degree is to restore competence of the LES while still allowing successful bolus transport into the stomach. A fundoplication procedure requires the reduction of any hiatal hernia, tightening of the diaphragmatic crura, return of an appropriate length of esophagus into the abdominal cavity, and increasing the pressure of the LES through the creation of a gastric fundoplication of the distal esophagus. These tasks may be accomplished by multiple approaches.

Thoracic Approach

The primary benefit of the thoracic approach is that it allows virgin access to the gastroesophageal junction (GEJ) in patients having undergone multiple or complicated prior abdominal surgeries. The trans-thoracic fundoplication is accomplished through a thoracotomy or video-assisted thoracoscopic surgery via the left chest. In this procedure, the mid to distal esophagus is mobilized, hiatal hernia is reduced, a partial 270° fundoplication is performed, and the hiatus is closed. An esophageal lengthening procedure may occasionally be required.

Open Abdominal Approach

With the proliferation of complex laparoscopic skills, rarely is an open approach to fundoplication indicated outside of the complex reoperation with prohibitive adhesive disease, on occasion of an indication for fundoplication coexisting with an independent indication for laparotomy or in a patient who will not tolerate laparoscopy.

Laparoscopic Abdominal Approach

The preferred and most common approach to accomplishing both primary and redo fundoplication is the laparoscopic approach. Not only does a laparoscopic approach result in less pain, but it facilitates earlier return to function and discharge and is more economical.[6] The real benefit of laparoscopic surgery is that it allows better and more complete visualization of the hiatus, GEJ, and posterior mediastinum than an open abdominal or thoracic approach. The CO_2 pneumoperitoneum also aids in the reduction of the hiatal hernia from the thorax, and if the pleura are violated during hernia reduction, the resulting pneumothorax rarely if ever requires a painful tube thoracostomy. Any of the variety of anterior or posterior partial or complete anterior fundoplication procedures may be accomplished by this approach depending on motility, associated anatomy, and procedures and surgeon or patient preference.

Robotic Fundoplication

Although a robotic approach to fundoplication has been described, we have not found a place for it in the practice of an advanced laparoscopic surgeon. Indications and limitations parallel those of laparoscopy.

Redo Antireflux Surgery

Redo antireflux surgery is frequently considered in the face of a disrupted or failed gastric fundoplication or recurrent hiatal hernia. The same diagnostic studies as indicated for first-time surgery are indicated before a second or redo fundoplication surgery, particularly if a significant amount of time has passed. Operative notes from the previous surgeries are helpful, as they can describe if any and what type of mesh may have been placed at the hiatus. Serious consideration of referral to an experienced foregut surgical specialist should be considered by those who are not familiar with the difficulty of redo surgery at the hiatus and in any patient who had prior mesh placement at the hiatus.

DIVERTING PROCEDURES FOR THE TREATMENT OF REFLUX DISEASE

The Roux-en-Y gastric bypass (RYGB) treats GERD through a different strategy than procedures augmenting the GEJ. Rather than retarding the reflux of caustic enteric and gastric secretions, the RYGB diverts the secretions from their origin into the more distal enteric tract. RYGB should be considered in several population of patients: (1) those with a body mass index of greater than 35 kg/m^2 owing to their high rates (31%) of failure after fundoplication surgery,[7] (2) those with very poor or absent esophageal motility, (3) those previously having complicated fundoplication surgery not amenable to redo, and (4) those with a history of sleeve gastrectomy with intractable reflux.

ELECTRICAL AUGMENTATION OF THE LOWER ESOPHAGEAL SPHINCTER

Currently undergoing Food and Drug Administration (FDA) trials after approval in Europe and South America is the EndoStim System (EndoStim, St. Louis, MO). This device consists of a pacemaker-type generator that is implanted in a subcutaneous pocket in the abdominal wall with 2 implantable bipolar electrodes that are sutured superficially through the muscular layer of the distal esophagus approximately 1 cm apart. The device generates a periodic electrical charge between the electrodes, stimulating the LES and increasing resting sphincter tone.[8] The device can be programmed by the physician in clinic, as would be a cardiac pacemaker device. The device battery is expected to last between 7 and 10 years depending on device type and use, at which time the battery may be changed during an outpatient surgical procedure.

Two trials have been published on the system. Results of the 2 published trials show similar efficacy.[9,10] The larger trial is multicenter and multinational with 44 patients followed to 6 months with incidence of pH <4.0 reduced from 10.0% to 3.8% after 3 months and to 4.4% at 6 months (P = .0001). Complications have been reported, including bowel injury during placement, and erosion and dysphagia in cases of simultaneous hiatal hernia repair.[10]

The EndoStim may in time prove to be a reasonable therapy in patients with impaired motility, inability to tolerate a prolonged or major operation, or other contraindication for alternative antireflux surgery or as a less invasive therapy for patients not desiring more invasive antireflux surgery who demonstrate only a partial response to pharmacologic therapy.[11] Studies are not available on long-term efficacy, impact on metaplasia, or the rate of recurrence of a hiatal hernia repaired at the time of implantation. We would advise caution in the implantation of this device in the setting of simultaneous hiatal hernia repair (**Box 1**, **Fig. 1**).

Box 1
Enrollment criteria for ongoing EndoStim device trial (NCT02749071)

Inclusion criteria

- Age 22 to 75

- Gastroesophageal reflux disease (GERD) symptoms of 6 months duration that are not completely treated with medical therapy

- Documented symptomatic improvement on medical therapy

- Documented excessive esophageal acid exposure off of medical therapy

- Esophagitis ≤ Los Angeles Grade B

- Adequate esophageal body contraction amplitude (>30 mm Hg for 30% of swallows and 30% peristaltic contraction on high-resolution manometry, or ≥30% peristaltic contraction with distal contractile index >450

- Suitable surgical candidates

Key exclusion criteria

- Previous procedure for GERD

- Hiatal hernia >3 cm as determined by endoscopy

- Esophageal stricture or significant dysmotility

Data from EndoStim Inc. An investigation on the EndoStim lower esophageal sphincter (LES) stimulation system for the treatment of reflux. In U.S. National Library of Medicine, Clinicaltrial.gov. Available at: https://clinicaltrials.gov/ct2/show/NCT02749071/. Accessed January 26, 2018.

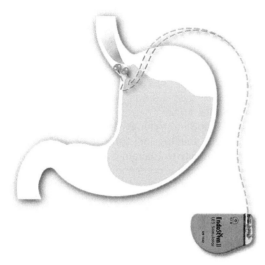

Fig. 1. EndosStim generator with leads attached. Figure illustrating placement of leads 1 cm apart at the GEJ. (©2018 EndoGastric Solutions, Inc. Redmond, WA, USA.)

MAGNETIC SPHINCTER AUGMENTATION DEVICE

The magnetic sphincter augmentation device (MSA) is indicated as an alternative to the complete gastric (Nissen) fundoplication. The device consists of a band of rare earth magnets that are encased in titanium, each of which is connected with a discontinuous segment of titanium wire to the adjacent beads. When closed around the GEJ, the MSA device increases the yield pressure of the LES/GEJ preventing pathologic reflux while still allowing the passage of solid or liquid bolus without inducting dysphagia and allowing the retrograde passage of gas and vomit, preventing gas-bloat or intractable retching sometimes so troublesome to those having undergone complete fundoplication.

Studies on the initial cohort of patients in a multicenter trial seeking FDA device approval showed excellent outcomes after MSA device implantation; 93% of patients will reduce proton pump inhibitor dosing by at least 50%, and decrease in esophagitis from 40% to 12% with high patient satisfaction.[12] Follow-up of this cohort at 5 years with 85% (85/100) continued to show cessation or significant reduction (>50%) in 90% of patients.[12] There was also a significant reduction in the prevalence and significance of esophagitis.

The placement of a foreign body in any part of the body, particularly near soft tissue is a proposal requiring careful consideration. Device erosion has been rare in initial studies at 0.2%, and was 0.1% in the analysis of the first 1000 cases reported in the literature.[13–15] The primary concerning

outcome after MSA implantation is dysphagia. In initial studies, the preoperative dysphagia rate was 6%. Postoperatively the rates of dysphagia in the immediate postoperative, 1-year, and 5-year time points was 68%, 11%, and 5%, respectively. In this study 19 (19%) of 100 patients required dilatation during the postoperative year.[16]

We believe that the incidence of dysphagia can be minimized through careful attention to not undersizing the device at time of implantation and careful patient selection, with a mind to the fact that patients with prominent atypical symptoms, particularly nausea and vomiting or laryngeal/pharyngeal symptoms, especially those with a potential psychiatric component, should be considered carefully and preoperative studies examined strictly before consideration of MSA implantation in the face of any concern. However, the duration of most dysphagia is short and with thorough preoperative counseling, well tolerated by most patients. It is important to make it clear to patients that for several days to weeks after surgery they will predictably experience mild dysphagia that typically resolves.

There is also growing evidence that the MSA device can be successfully used simultaneously in the treatment of hiatal hernia of at least 7 cm in size. We recently published a study of 47 patients with 89% follow-up at 19 months with 89% of patients remaining off pharmacologic therapy and only a 4.3% recurrence rate.[17] Further study on the success and safety of the MSA in more complex situations, including implantation at the time of large hiatal hernia repair, after failed fundoplication with intact wrap, and in patients with reflux following sleeve gastrectomy is needed, and ongoing by our group and others (**Box 2**, **Fig. 2**).

Box 2
Indications and contraindication for LINX magnetic sphincter augmentation

Indications

- Patients who seek an alternative to continuous medical acid suppression therapy to treat the symptoms of GERD.

Key contraindications

- Allergy to titanium, stainless steel, ferrous metals, or nickel
- Likely or known need for MRI scan in a machine of greater than 0.7 to 1.5 T depending on generation of magnetic sphincter augmentation device

Data from Torax Medical Inc. Indication, safety and warnings [Linx]. In: Commercial Linx Web site. Available at: http://www.linxforlife.com/abridged-statement. Accessed January 26, 2018.

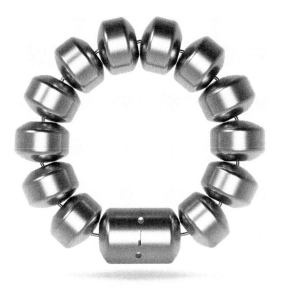

Fig. 2. The LINX device consists of a variable number of titanium beads each encasing a rare earth magnet. The device provides dynamic and static augmentation of the LES yield. (*Courtesy of* Torax Medical, Shoreview, MN. Available at: http://www.linxforlife.com/dist/images/linx-device-full-closed-grey.jpg; with permission.)

SUMMARY

A multitude of extraluminal therapies exist for GERD. The choice of the correct procedure should depend as much on the surgeon's expertise as patient preference. In a patient with no prior surgical intervention, the gold standard remains a fundoplication. In these straightforward patients there is now sufficient evidence to recommend an MSA if placed by a surgeon with experience in the procedure as well as its postoperative management. The MSA offers similar reflux control when compared with the Nissen with the added benefit of retained ability to vomit and belch with the potential for better long-term (10 yr+) results; however, this has yet to be shown. The Toupet procedure remains a viable option for both those with or without impaired esophageal motility.

Looking to the future, we suspect that the EndoStim may find a place in the treatment of GERD; what that place is remains unclear at the present time. An area of growing interest is the treatment of GERD following sleeve gastrectomy. We believe that the MSA device may prove of particular utility in this clinical situation, as may revision to RYGB.

REFERENCES

1. Garg SK, Gurusamy KS. Laparoscopic fundoplication surgery versus medical management for gastro-oesophageal reflux disease (GORD) in adults. Cochrane Database Syst Rev 2015;(11): 1–53.
2. Mittal RK, Balaban DH. The esophagogastric junction. N Engl J Med 1997;13:924–32.
3. Kahrilas PH, Lin S, Chen J, et al. The effect of hiatus hernia on gastro-oesophageal junction pressure. Gut 1999;4:476–82.
4. Tatum JM, Samakar K, Bowdish ME, et al. Videoesophagography vs. endoscopy for prediction of intraoperative hiatal hernia size. Am Surg 2018; 84(3):387–91.
5. Holloway RH, Dent J. Pathophysiology of gastroesophageal reflux. Lower esophageal sphincter dysfunction in gastroesophageal reflux disease. Gastroenterol Clin North Am 1990;19: 517–35.
6. Richards KF, Fisher KS, Flores JH, et al. Laparoscopic Nissen fundoplication: cost, morbidity, and outcomes compared with open surgery. Surg Laparosc Endosc 1996;2:140–3.
7. Perex AR, Moncure AC, Rattner DW. Obesity adversely affects the outcome of antireflux surgery. Surg Endosc 2001;9:986–9.
8. Crowell MD. Implanted electrical devices and gastroesophageal reflux disease: an effective approach to treatment. Expert Rev Gastroenterol Hepatol 2013;3:189–91.
9. Rodriguez L, Rodriquez P, Gomex B, et al. Long-term results of electrical stimulation of the lower esophageal sphincter for the treatment of gastroesophageal reflux disease. Endoscopy 2015;8: 595–604.
10. Kappelle WF, Bredenoord AJ, Conchillo JM, et al. Electrical stimulation therapy of the lower esophageal sphincter for refractory gatro-oesophageal reflux disease—interm results of an international multicenter trial. Aliment Pharmacol Ther 2015;5: 614–25.
11. Soffer E, Rodriquez L, Rordriguez P, et al. Effect of electrical stimulation of the lower esophageal sphincter in gastroesophageal reflux disease patients refractory to proton pump inhibitors. World J Gastrointest Pharmacol Ther 2016;1: 145–55.
12. Ganz RA, Peters JH, Horgan S, et al. Esophageal sphincter device for gastroesophageal reflux disease. N Engl J Med 2013;368:719–27.
13. Lipham JC, Taiganides PA, Louie BE, et al. Safety analysis of first 1000 patients treated with magnetic sphincter augmentation for gastroesophageal reflux disease. Dis Esophagus 2015;4: 305–11.
14. Bielefeldt K. Adverse events after implantation of a magnetic sphincter augmentation device for gastroesophageal reflux. Clin Gastroenterol Hepatol 2016; 10:1507–8.

15. Asti E, Siboni S, Lazzari V, et al. Removal of the magnetic sphincter augmentation device. Ann Surg 2016;265:941–5.

16. Ganz RA, Edmundowicz SA, Taiganides PA, et al. Long-term outcomes of patients receiving a magnetic sphincter augmentation device for gastroesophageal reflux. Clin Gastroenterol Hepatol 2016;5:671–7.

17. Rona KA, Tatum JM, Zehetner J. Hiatal hernia recurrence following magnetic sphincter augmentation and posterior cruroplasty: intermediate-term outcomes. Surg Endosc 2018;32(7):3374–9.

Endoluminal Approaches to Gastroesophageal Reflux Disease

Marissa Anne Mayor, MD[a],
Hiran Chrishantha Fernando, MBBS, FRCS, FRCSEd[b],*

KEYWORDS

• Endoluminal • GERD • Endoscopic • TIF (transoral incisionless fundoplication) • Stretta

KEY POINTS

• Endoluminal therapies are attractive minimally invasive options for the treatment of GERD, although long-term data are lacking further than 5 to 7 years.
• Stretta (radiofrequency ablation) controls reflux activity by decreasing the response rate and compliance of the lower esophageal sphincter, and is approximately 50% effective in reducing proton pump inhibitor (PPI) use.
• Endoluminal fundoplication (EsophyX or MUSE devices) is also approximately 50% effective in reducing PPI use. Unlike Stretta, endoscopic fundoplication has been associated with normalization of esophageal acid exposure in approximately 50% of patients.

INTRODUCTION

Gastroesophageal reflux disease (GERD) is one of the most frequent diagnoses evaluated by gastroenterologists, with a prevalence of approximately 10% to 20% in Western countries.[1] The physiologic mechanism of the disease is multifactorial, and may be concurrent with variable combinations of decreased lower esophageal sphincter (LES) tone, hiatal herniation, esophageal dysmotility, and gastroparesis. An initial trial of nonoperative management with dietary and lifestyle modification in addition to an 8-week trial of proton pump inhibitors (PPIs) is first-line therapy. However, satisfactory symptom relief occurs in as few as 30% to 40% of patients and often requires lifelong PPI administration.[1] The Nissen fundoplication is the current gold standard for surgical management of GERD, and has been the mainstay for antireflux procedures[2,3]; however, the invasiveness of the procedure renders it less attractive to many patients, particularly those who have a more moderate symptom profile. Additionally, many patients are concerned about side effects of antireflux surgery, such as gas-bloat and difficulty with belching.[2,4] Endoluminal approaches were pioneered in the 1980s to address these, and recent advances in device design and technique have generated renewed interest.

BRIEF HISTORY OF ENDOLUMINAL THERAPIES

Two early endoluminal fundoplication devices were the Endocinch (Bard, Murray Hill, NJ) and the NDO-plicator (NDO Surgical, Mansfield, MA). The Endocinch was the first endoscopic fundoplication device and functioned by plicating the mucosa.[5] This device was taken off the market after long-term follow-up failed to demonstrate

Disclosure Statement: The authors have nothing to disclose.
[a] Department of Surgery, INOVA Fairfax Medical Campus, 3300 Gallows Road-NPT 2nd Floor, Falls Church, VA 22042, USA; [b] Thoracic Oncology, Department of Surgery, INOVA Fairfax Medical Campus, 3300 Gallows Road-NPT 2nd Floor, Falls Church, VA 22042, USA
* Corresponding author.
E-mail address: hiran.fernando@inova.org

Thorac Surg Clin 28 (2018) 527–532
https://doi.org/10.1016/j.thorsurg.2018.07.008
1547-4127/18/© 2018 Elsevier Inc. All rights reserved.

improvement in symptoms.[6] The NDO-plicator was developed as a full-thickness plicating device, designed to conduct a single plication in the cardia using polytetrafluoroethylene-pledgeted suture. Three-year follow-up demonstrated a PPI cessation rate of 59% with improvement in symptoms in 55% of patients.[7] However, this device has since been taken off the market and is no longer available. Another strategy applied endoscopically to the treatment of GERD has been enhancement of LES tone using various injections. The Enteryx used a biopolymer injected into the muscle layer of the LES.[8] This was removed from the market after several complications (including 1 death) secondary to poor localization of the injection.[9] These complications led to decreased interest in endoluminal therapies using the same strategy as the Enteryx, such as the Gatekeeper device (injection of hydrophilic material)[10] or Teflon injection.[11]

The 2 categories of devices for endoluminal therapy currently on the market are the Stretta device (radiofrequency ablation) and endoluminal fundoplication devices (the EsophyX and MUSE devices) and are described in detail later in this article.

CURRENT GOLD STANDARD: NISSEN FUNDOPLICATION

The gold standard for surgical management of GERD is the laparoscopic Nissen fundoplication,[12] which is the benchmark for endoscopic therapies (for more detail, please see section 4 by Lipham and colleagues). The overall success rate as measured by resolution of reflux symptoms off PPIs ranges from 80% to 96%[2,13–15]; however, fundoplication may be complicated by long-term dysphagia.[4,13,16–18] Additionally, patients may complain of gas-bloat in 15% to 50% and difficulty with belching in 14% to 70%.[4,16] Finally, the invasive nature of the procedure makes it a less attractive therapeutic modality.

CURRENT ENDOSCOPIC THERAPIES
Stretta

The Stretta system (Mederi Therapeutics Inc., Norwalk, CT) applies radiofrequency ablation to the LES using a balloon catheter assembly. After confirming the location of the squamo-columnar junction, the catheter is positioned within 1.0 to 1.5 cm proximal to this, and the balloon inflated. When activated, the system applies radiofrequency energy through 4 needle tips projecting at 90° from the balloon. The balloon is deflated and the catheter rotated approximately 45° and additional ablation performed at the same level. A series of

ablations is then performed progressing distally and below the squamo-columnar junction. The resultant nerve ablation, fibrosis, and increase in wall thickness controls reflux activity by decreasing the response rate and compliance of the LES.[19–21] This system has been approved by the Food and Drug Administration since 2001 and has the advantage of several trials with long-term follow-up.[22] Several recent meta-analyses have examined the clinical outcomes of the Stretta system with mixed results.[23–25] The most recent of these by Fass and colleagues[25] pooled 2468 patients from 4 randomized controlled trials (RCTs), 23 cohort studies, and 1 registry. Outcomes evaluated in the meta-analysis were both subjective (PPI use, GERD health-related quality of life [HRQL], heartburn score) and objective (presence of erosive esophagitis, esophageal acid exposure, LES basal pressure). The investigators found a significant reduction in the use of PPIs after Stretta therapy, with less than half of baseline PPI users still using PPIs (relative risk 0.49, n = 850/1743). Both GERD-HRQL and heartburn scores significantly improved after Stretta treatment in comparison with sham treatments. The investigators also reported a statistically significant improvement in both erosive esophagitis and esophageal acid exposure, although there was significant heterogeneity among the included studies. There was no statistically significant improvement in the LES basal pressure after pooled estimate.

Notably, the Stretta approach has demonstrated long-term durability. The 10-year follow-up of an open-label clinical trial reported normalization of GERD-HQRL scores in 72% of 217 patients.[22] Forty-one percent of patients had maintained complete cessation of PPIs at the 10-year mark, with 64% reporting a 50% or greater reduction in PPI use. Interestingly, of 33 patients who began the study with Barrett metaplasia, 28 had complete resolution on follow-up endoscopy.

An additional advantage to the Stretta procedure is that it does not preclude further therapy; should treatment fail, a laparoscopic fundoplication may still be performed. It can also be used as an adjunct for failures after fundoplication.[26]

Endoscopic Fundoplication

Currently there are 2 devices on the market for performance of endoscopic fundoplication: the EsophyX (Endogastric Solutions, Redmond, WA) and the MUSE (Medigus Ltd., Omer, Israel) systems. The EsophyX creates a 270-degree wrap using a pin and suction technique (**Fig. 1**). The EsophyX device is passed through the esophagus alongside the endoscope and retroflexed in the

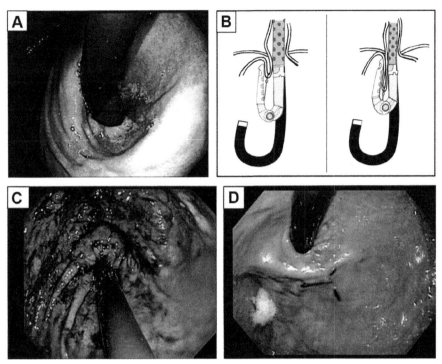

Fig. 1. Representative case and graphic representation of endoscopic fundoplication. (*A*) Retroflexed view of the esophago-gastric junction (EGJ) demonstrating Hill grade III defect. (*B*) The helical retractor of the EsophyX device (Endogastric Solutions, Redmond, WA, USA) is used to pull the EGJ into the device. (*C*) Immediate result post-procedure; (*D*) Results at 4-week follow-up.

stomach under direct vision, after endoscopic retroflexion. The device is then rotated to the 11 o'clock position and slightly opened. The fastening portion of the device, the helical retractor, is positioned onto the gastroesophageal junction on the esophageal side and traction is placed to pull the junction into the device. The device is then closed and 4 or more polypropylene fasteners are deployed to secure the plication. This step is repeated at the 1 o'clock position. Fasteners are then deployed at the 5 and 7 o'clock positions at a deeper level, resulting in an approximately 2-cm partial fundoplication.

We recently reported on the long-term follow-up of 41 patients who had undergone the transoral incisionless fundoplication (TIF) procedure using the EsophyX device.[27] At an average of 24-month follow-up, there was a significant improvement in the GERD-HRQL. Cessation of PPI use was observed in 44% of the 39 patients who had initially been on PPIs and had longer than 6-month follow-up. Testoni and colleagues[28] recently reported their 6-year follow-up of patients undergoing TIF, and demonstrated a decreased use or cessation of PPIs in 84% of patients. The most recent meta-analysis pooled data from 5 RCTs and 13 prospective observational studies.[29] The

investigators demonstrated a decrease in the total number of refluxes despite no significant difference in the esophageal acid exposure time. PPIs were resumed in most patients, albeit at a reduced dose. The overall complication rate was 2.4% and included perforation and bleeding. Notably, there have been no reports of post-TIF gas-bloat symptoms, which may be a complication of Nissen fundoplication.[30,31] Although the meta-analysis did not demonstrate a significant improvement in esophageal acid exposure, several studies including a multicenter randomized trial comparing TIF to best medical therapy demonstrated normalization of acid exposure in 54% of patients.[31]

The MUSE system is a newer device that functions similarly to the EsophyX but uses an endoscopic stapler. Currently there are only a few reports with this device. A pilot study reported on 13 patients with 5-year follow-up, demonstrating improvement in the GERD-related symptom score and a complete PPI cessation rate of 54%.[32] One additional multicenter study demonstrated a 64.6% PPI cessation rate among 66 patients with a mean 6-month follow-up.[33] This study also demonstrated a significant improvement in the GERD-HRQL scores.

Table 1
Comparison of Nissen, Stretta, and endoluminal fundoplication

	Nissen	Stretta	Endoluminal Fundoplication
PPI cessation rate, %	80–96	29–86	63–86
Healing of erosive esophagitis, %	93	85	86
Normalization of esophageal acid exposure time, %	93	20–22	37–89
Duration of follow-up	Up to 17 y; multiple high-quality trials with 5–10-y follow-up	Up to 10 y; most 2–5-y follow-up	Up to 5–6 y; Most 2–3-y follow-up
References	2–4,12,18,35	20,22,23,25,26	27,28,30,31,34

Variability in outcomes with endoscopic fundoplication procedures may be due to patient selection. Factors found to be associated with improved success include hiatal hernia <2 cm and normal esophageal motility.[30,34] However, patients with impaired motility are more likely to have a poorer outcome with a more standard laparoscopic fundoplication, so a less aggressive endoscopic repair may be a good option for such patients. Another consideration is that the EsophyX device

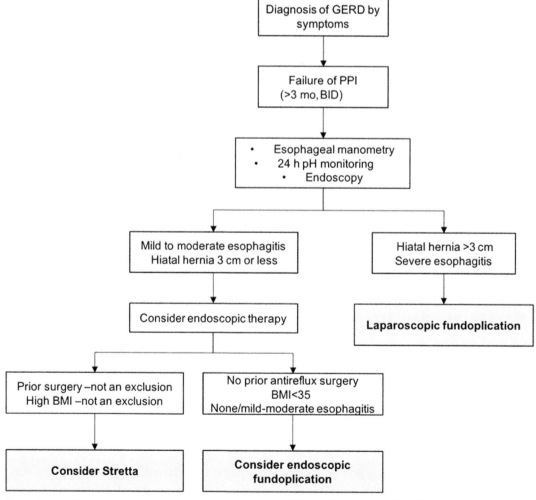

Fig. 2. Proposed algorithm for endoluminal management of GERD. BID, twice a day; BMI, body mass index.

has undergone several recent improvements, and more studies are needed to evaluate this and the MUSE device with long-term follow-up.

CONCLUDING STATEMENTS

Endoscopic therapies for the management of GERD have made significant advances in the past 20 years. Both the Stretta procedure and the TIF procedure provide alternatives to the more invasive laparoscopic Nissen fundoplication. The complication rate of either procedure is low. Overall PPI cessation rates are approximately half that seen in patients who have undergone the Nissen fundoplication. Quality of life improvement is seen in roughly three-quarters of patients, compared with the greater than 90% rate seen with the Nissen (**Table 1**). Additionally, long-term outcomes have not been reported in comparison with some reports with 10 or more years of follow-up after laparoscopic fundoplication.[35] Patient selection is key, with endoscopic therapies being ideal for patients without a large hiatal hernia (**Fig. 2**). As more long-term data become available, endoscopic therapies will play a critical role in the management of GERD.

REFERENCES

1. Katz PO, Gerson LB, Vela MF. Guidelines for the diagnosis and management of gastroesophageal reflux disease. Am J Gastroenterol 2013;108(3):308–28.
2. Peters JH, DeMeester TR, Crookes P, et al. The treatment of gastroesophageal reflux disease with laparoscopic Nissen fundoplication: prospective evaluation of 100 patients with "typical" symptoms. Ann Surg 1998;228(1):40–50. Available at: http://www.pubmedcentral.nih.gov/articlerender.fcgi?artid=1191426&tool=pmcentrez&rendertype=abstract.
3. Streets CG, DeMeester SR, DeMeester TR, et al. Excellent quality of life after Nissen fundoplication depends on successful elimination of reflux symptoms and not the invasiveness of the surgical approach. Ann Thorac Surg 2002;74(4):1019–25.
4. Rantanen TK, Salo JA, Salminen JT. Functional outcome after laparoscopic or open Nissen fundoplication: a follow-up study. Arch Surg 1999;134(3):240–4. Available at: http://ovidsp.ovid.com/ovidweb.cgi?T=JS&PAGE=reference&D=emed7&NEWS=N&AN=29136005.
5. Kadirkamanathan SS, Evans DF, Gong F, et al. Antireflux operations at flexible endoscopy using endoluminal stitching techniques: An experimental study. Gastrointest Endosc 1996;44(2):133–43.
6. Schiefke I, Zabel-Langhennig A, Neumann S, et al. Long term failure of endoscopic gastroplication (EndoCinch). Gut 2005;54(6):752–8.
7. Pleskow D, Rothstein R, Kozarek R, et al. Endoscopic full-thickness plication for the treatment of GERD: five-year long-term multicenter results. Surg Endosc 2008;22(2):326–32.
8. Deviére J, Pastorelli A, Louis H, et al. Endoscopic implantation of a biopolymer in the lower esophageal sphincter for gastroesophageal reflux: a pilot study. Gastrointest Endosc 2002;55(3):335–41.
9. Wong RF, Davis TV, Peterson KA. Complications involving the mediastinum after injection of Enteryx for GERD. Gastrointest Endosc 2005;61(6):753–6.
10. Fockens P, Bruno MJ, Gabbrielli A, et al. Endoscopic augmentation of the lower esophageal sphincter for the treatment of gastroesophageal reflux disease: multicenter study of the Gatekeeper Reflux Repair System. Endoscopy 2004;36(8):682–9.
11. Feretis C, Benakis P, Dimopoulos C, et al. Endoscopic implantation of Plexiglas (PMMA) microspheres for the treatment of GERD. Gastrointest Endosc 2001;53(4):423–6.
12. DeMeester TR, Bonavina L, Albertucci M. Nissen fundoplication for gastroesophageal reflux disease. Evaluation of primary repair in 100 consecutive patients. Ann Surg 1986;204(1):9–20.
13. Hunter JG, Swanstrom L, Waring JP. Dysphagia after laparoscopic antireflux surgery. The impact of operative technique. Ann Surg 1996;224(1):51–7.
14. Hinder RA, Filipi CJ, Wetscher G, et al. Laparoscopic Nissen fundoplication is an effective treatment for gastroesophageal reflux disease. Ann Surg 1994;220(4):472–3.
15. Weerts JM, Dallemagne B, Hamoir E, et al. Laparoscopic Nissen fundoplication: detailed analysis of 132 patients. Surg Laparosc Endosc 1993;3(5):359–64. Available at: http://www.ncbi.nlm.nih.gov/entrez/query.fcgi?cmd=Retrieve&db=PubMed&dopt=Citation&list_uids=8261262.
16. Tian ZC, Wang B, Shan CX, et al. A meta-analysis of randomized controlled trials to compare long-term outcomes of Nissen and Toupet fundoplication for gastroesophageal reflux disease. PLoS One 2015;10(6):e0127627.
17. Koch OO, Kaindlstorfer A, Antoniou SA, et al. Comparison of results from a randomized trial 1 year after laparoscopic Nissen and Toupet fundoplications. Surg Endosc 2013;27(7):2383–90.
18. Oor JE, Roks DJ, Broeders JA, et al. Seventeen-year outcome of a randomized clinical trial comparing laparoscopic and conventional Nissen fundoplication. Ann Surg 2017;266(1):23–8.
19. Kim MS, Holloway RH, Dent J, et al. Radiofrequency energy delivery to the gastric cardia inhibits triggering of transient lower esophageal sphincter relaxation and gastroesophageal reflux in dogs. Gastrointest Endosc 2003;57(1):17–22.
20. Tam WCE. Delivery of radiofrequency energy to the lower oesophageal sphincter and gastric cardia

inhibits transient lower oesophageal sphincter relaxations and gastro-oesophageal reflux in patients with reflux disease. Gut 2003;52(4):479–85.

21. Corley DA, Katz P, Wo JM, et al. Improvement of gastroesophageal reflux symptoms after radiofrequency energy: a randomized, sham-controlled trial. Gastroenterology 2003;125(3):668–76.

22. Noar M, Squires P, Noar E, et al. Long-term maintenance effect of radiofrequency energy delivery for refractory GERD: a decade later. Surg Endosc 2014;28(8):2323–33.

23. Perry K. A., Banerjee A, Melvin WS. Radiofrequency energy delivery to the lower esophageal sphincter reduces esophageal acid exposure and improves GERD symptoms: a systematic review and meta-analysis [review]. Surg Laparosc Endosc Percutan Tech 2012;22(4):283–8.

24. Lipka S, Kumar A, Richter JE. No evidence for efficacy of radiofrequency ablation for treatment of gastroesophageal reflux disease: a systematic review and meta-analysis. Clin Gastroenterol Hepatol 2015;13(6):1058–67.e1.

25. Fass R, Cahn F, Scotti DJ, et al. Systematic review and meta-analysis of controlled and prospective cohort efficacy studies of endoscopic radiofrequency for treatment of gastroesophageal reflux disease. Surg Endosc 2017; 31(12):4865–82.

26. Noar M, Squires P, Khan S. Radiofrequency energy delivery to the lower esophageal sphincter improves gastroesophageal reflux patient-reported outcomes in failed laparoscopic Nissen fundoplication cohort. Surg Endosc 2017;31(7):2854–62.

27. Ebright M, Sridhar P, Litle VR, et al. Endoscopic fundoplication effectiveness for controlling symptoms of gastroesophageal reflux disease. Innovations (Phila) 2017;12(3):180–5.

28. Testoni PA, Testoni S, Mazzoleni G, et al. Long-term efficacy of transoral incisionless fundoplication with Esophyx (TIF 2.0) and factors affecting outcomes in GERD patients followed for up to 6 years: a prospective single-center study. Surg Endosc 2015; 29(9):2770–80.

29. Huang X, Chen S, Zhao H, et al. Efficacy of transoral incisionless fundoplication (TIF) for the treatment of GERD: a systematic review with meta-analysis. Surg Endosc 2017;31(3):1032–44.

30. Testoni PA, Mazzoleni G, Testoni SGG. Transoral incisionless fundoplication for gastro-esophageal reflux disease: techniques and outcomes. World J Gastrointest Pharmacol Ther 2016;7(2):179.

31. Trad KS, Fox MA, Simoni G, et al. Transoral fundoplication offers durable symptom control for chronic GERD: 3-year report from the TEMPO randomized trial with a crossover arm. Surg Endosc 2017; 31(6):2498–508.

32. Roy-Shapira A, Bapaye A, Date S, et al. Trans-oral anterior fundoplication: 5-year follow-up of pilot study. Surg Endosc 2015;29(12):3717–21.

33. Zacherl J, Roy-Shapira A, Bonavina L, et al. Endoscopic anterior fundoplication with the Medigus Ultrasonic Surgical Endostapler (MUSE) for gastroesophageal reflux disease: 6-month results from a multi-center prospective trial. Surg Endosc 2015;29(1):220–9.

34. Fernando HC. Endoscopic fundoplication: patient selection and technique. J Vis Surg 2017;3:121.

35. Broeders JA, Rijnhart-de Jong HG, Draaisma WA, et al. Ten-year outcome of laparoscopic and conventional Nissen fundoplication. Ann Surg 2009;250(5): 698–706.

Management of the Difficult Hiatal Hernia

Matthew Rochefort, MD[a], Jon O. Wee, MD[b],*

KEYWORDS

- Paraesophageal hernia • Mesh • Gastroplasty • Fundoplication

KEY POINTS

- Repair of the hernias requires assessment of the esophageal length and crural tension.
- Shortened esophageal length can be address with aggressive esophageal mobilization, but may require a lengthening procedure.
- Mesh reinforcement of the hiatus can result in short term benefit, but may not improve long term outcomes.

A hiatal hernia refers to the herniation of an intra-abdominal organ or organs into the thoracic cavity through the space between the left and right crus of the diaphragm. The vast majority of hiatal hernias are referred to as type I or sliding hernias. In this situation, weakness of the phrenoesophageal ligament allows herniation of the gastroesophageal junction into the thoracic cavity thereby bringing the cardia of the stomach above the diaphragmatic hiatus. A type II hiatal hernia is a paraesophageal hernia in which the gastroesophageal junction is fixed and another portion of the stomach herniates through the diaphragmatic hiatus into the chest alongside the esophagus. A type III hernia is a combination of type I and II whereby both the gastroesophageal junction and another portion of the stomach have herniated through the diaphragmatic hiatus. A type IV hiatal hernia indicates that an intra-abdominal organ in addition to the stomach has herniated through the hiatus, commonly the colon or the small bowel but may include the spleen or pancreas.

Type I or sliding hiatal hernias are becoming increasingly common, likely due to the increasing incidence of obesity; however, they usually require operative intervention only if they become symptomatic, as in conjunction with an antireflux procedure. Type II-IV hiatal hernias are commonly repaired once identified because of the concern for acute gastric volvulus and catastrophic strangulation of the stomach,[1,2] in addition to symptom correction, such as postprandial chest discomfort, dysphagia, or reflux. Acute presentations can lead to the need for emergency detorsion and a well-documented increased morbidity and mortality compared with elective laparoscopic repair. It is estimated that the risk of serious complication due to the presence of a paraesophageal hiatal hernia is approximately 1% per year.[3] Type III-IV together have been referred to as "giant paraesophageal hernias," whereby at least 30% of the stomach is contained within the thoracic cavity,[4] and the surgical management of this clinical situation is the focus of this review.

SURGICAL TREATMENT OF HIATAL HERNIAS

The history of operative repair of hiatal hernias begins in the early twentieth century, when open abdominal laparotomy incisions were used to

Disclosure: Dr M. Rochefort has nothing to disclose. Dr J.O. Wee is a consultant for Medtronic.
[a] Division of Thoracic Surgery, Brigham & Women's Hospital, 75 Francis Street, Boston, MA 02115, USA;
[b] Esophageal Surgery, Division of Thoracic Surgery, Brigham & Women's Hospital, 75 Francis Street, Boston, MA 02115, USA
* Corresponding author.
E-mail address: jwee@bwh.harvard.edu

Thorac Surg Clin 28 (2018) 533–539
https://doi.org/10.1016/j.thorsurg.2018.07.001
1547-4127/18/© 2018 Elsevier Inc. All rights reserved.

gain access to the esophageal hiatus. At that time, the openings in the diaphragmatic hiatus were closed directly around the organs that naturally passed through, namely the esophagus.[5] During the second half of the twentieth century, the focus transitioned to procedures performed through the thoracic cavity whereby the hernia sac could be reduced into the abdomen, the diaphragmatic opening could be narrowed under direct vision, and extensive mobilization of the esophagus could be performed. The subsequent development of the fundoplication and the ability to treat reflux disease by wrapping the stomach around the distal esophagus led to the broad incorporation of a fundoplication as an integral portion of repair of a paraesophageal hernia.[5]

The advent of minimally invasive surgery has dramatically increased the number of reflux and hiatal hernia operations being performed. Laparoscopy provides improved visualization of the hiatus, dissection of the esophagus and the hernia sac can be performed well up into the mediastinum under direct vision, and is associated with a significantly shorter length of stay, less need of a nasogastric tube in place, less postoperative pain, and decreased morbidity compared with open repairs.[6] However laparoscopic repairs have higher reported recurrence rates. In one highly quoted study out of the University of Southern California, the rate of radiologic recurrences following laparoscopic suture cruroplasty repair for paraesophageal hernias was 42%.[7] Possible reasons include decreased adhesion generation following laparoscopy, less meticulous mediastinal dissection of the hernia sac, and less tactile feedback and recognition of crural closures under tension. As longer-term follow-up is available, it has also been demonstrated that the prevalence of hernia recurrence increases over time with greater long-term follow-up.[8,9]

RISK FACTOR FOR RECURRENCE

Some of the factors that contribute to the recurrence of hiatal hernias after repair include the dynamic nature of the esophageal hiatus, with continuous movement secondary to respiratory excursion, esophageal peristalsis, and cardiac activity, and the pressure gradient between the peritoneum and the thorax that is heightened during coughing or sneezing.[6,10] Any repair to a hernia defect in the hiatus is subject to 2 forms of tension. Axial tension is generated due to displacement of the gastroesophageal junction into the mediastinum. This displacement could be in response to an intrinsically shortened esophagus due to longitudinal collagen contraction resulting from

scarring and fibrosis secondary to repeated exposure of the distal esophagus to gastric contents.[4,11,12] With each swallow, the esophagus shortens and applies a constant force against the hiatal opening.[13] Radial tension is due to the chronic dilation of the hiatal opening and the force required to bring the edges of the crura back together. The crural pillars are also usually quite thin in large hernias and made of attenuated muscle fibers and not fascia that can lead to sutures pulling through when tied under tension.[6,10]

To address these 2 forms of tension, the surgical repair of hiatal hernias via a laparoscopic approach has some well-accepted tenets. These include thorough preoperative testing, meticulous atraumatic technique, routine division of the short gastric vessels, complete reduction and resection of the hernia sac, circumferential dissection of the esophagus up into the mediastinum to provide a 2-cm to 3-cm length of tension-free intra-abdominal esophagus, careful preservation of the vagus nerves, maintenance of the peritoneal lining covering the crura, posterior primary crural closure over a bougie, and an associated gastric fundoplication.[4,6,11,12,14–18] Preoperative planning includes a barium esophagram, upper endoscopy, and esophageal manometry, and for all patients with a significant component of gastroesophageal reflux, a pH probe.[16] The lack of complete reduction of the hernia sac from the mediastinum is associated with increased frequency of postoperative seroma formation and increased risk of recurrence of the hernia.[1,16] The addition of the fundoplication addresses the gastroesophageal reflux symptoms that most patients with giant paraesophageal hernias present with and theoretically helps to anchor the gastroesophageal junction below the level of the diaphragm.[1] Posterior suture cruroplasty is the preferred method of crural closure; however, occasional anterior sutures may be required to close the crural defect without inducing undue angulation of the esophagus as it passes through the hiatus.[13,16] In rare circumstances in which the preoperative manometry demonstrates a severe esophageal motility disorder, more than 90% of failed peristalsis, then a partial fundoplication may be favored to decrease the risk of postoperative dysphagia.[16] The addition of a fundoplication, although useful as an antireflux procedure, has not been proven to reduce the rate of reherniation following laparoscopic hernia repair.[19]

PERMANENT MESH

The advent of synthetic mesh and popularization of tension-free repair for inguinal and ventral hernias with demonstration of reduced recurrence led to the application of synthetic mesh reinforcement of hiatal hernia repairs.

Frantzides and colleagues,[20] from Rush, performed a randomized prospective study of mesh repair versus suture crural closure on 72 patients with hiatal hernias larger than 8 cm. In the prosthetic mesh group, they used an onlay of oval mesh with a radial defect that was used to form a "keyhole" around the esophagus. All of the patients received a 3-cm floppy Nissen fundoplication in additional to the crural closure. They found that at up to 6 years of follow-up there were no recurrences in the mesh group and there was a 22% recurrence rate in the simple cruroplasty group, and that all of the patients with radiographic recurrences were symptomatic.[20] They did not identify any patients with either stricture or erosion following repair with polytetrafluoroethylene (PTFE), but they acknowledge that repairs with polypropylene should be avoided given the risk for erosion at the hiatus. They concluded that the addition of the mesh is responsible for reducing the tension on the repair and therefore allows for improved healing.

Granderath and colleagues,[21] from Austria, performed a randomized control trial comparing simple cruroplasty following laparoscopic Nissen fundoplication to prosthetic closure with a polypropylene mesh. They similarly performed the mesh repair as an onlay but did not include the radial defect and did not encircle the esophagus with the mesh. The mesh was only placed posterior to the esophagus. They found that the rate of intrathoracic wrap migration in the group repaired with a prosthetic mesh was significantly less (1%) than the group with a simple cruroplasty (6%). They did notice a significantly higher rate of dysphagia in the patients with the prosthetic wrap at the 3-month time point; however, at 1-year follow-up, there was no longer a significant difference between the 2 groups. They surmised that with the mesh placed in the posterior position, it does not come in contact with the esophagus at all, but instead with the posterior portion of the fundic wrap, thereby providing some buffer to esophageal erosions.

Similarly, Muller-Stitch and colleagues,[22] from Switzerland, repaired 16 patients with a butterfly shaped mesh placed in the posterior location, and they noted that the rate of radiographic recurrence was reduced from 19% in the simple cruroplasty group to 0% in the mesh-reinforced group. The mesh used in these repairs was a combination of Prolene and Vicryl, which the group believed would reduce the potential for mesh-related complications. This study had a significant limitation in that the length of follow-up was significantly longer for patients with simple cruroplasty than for the mesh-reinforced repairs. In contrast to the group from Rush, they reported that only half of the radiographic recurrences were symptomatic, and that there was no significant difference in the symptomatic outcome between the mesh repair and the simple cruroplasty group.

Despite the positive results from these studies, there is still a significant hesitancy to place synthetic mesh during hiatal hernia repairs due to the potential for significant complications when placed near the dynamic esophageal hiatus, including the possibility of erosion, ulceration, stricture, and obstruction.[6,7,9,10,16,17] In a review of the complications associated with permanent mesh when placed at the hiatus, there were 6 patients who required an esophagectomy and an additional patient who required a gastrectomy to treat the complications of mesh erosion into the lumen.[10] It is thought that erosions occur from the constant movement of the esophagus against the solid edge of the mesh, with the mesh cutting into the esophagus over time. This happens even more frequently when the mesh is used to bridge the crural defect, as this results in increased contact between the esophagus and the mesh.[2,23] The other commonly reported complication was the creation of a dense band of fibrosis around the implanted prosthesis, which results in significant dysphagia.[10,18] These complications occurred over the course of months to years with an average time to complication of 23 months.

BIOLOGIC MESH

The concern over the relatively high recurrence rates associated with pure suture repair of the hiatus in conjunction with concern over potential complications associated with a permanent foreign material near the hiatus led to the investigation of biologic material reinforcement of the hiatus. Additional theoretic benefits of biologic mesh include resistance to infection if placed in a contaminated field, decreased inflammatory reaction, availability for neovascularization, and a reconstruction that ultimately is made of natural tissue.[6,24] For patients with large hiatal defects that cannot easily be closed without tension, the use of a small intestine submucosa and non–cross-linked human collagen matrix can be used to buttress the repair.[16]

Oelschlager and colleagues[6] performed a multi-center prospective randomized trial, of patients with type II-IV paraesophageal hernias, comparing suture closure of the hiatus to suture closure of the hiatus reinforced with a U-shaped piece of porcine small intestinal submucosa (Cook Surgical, Bloomington, IN). The mesh was used to buttress the posterior hiatal closure and the limbs extended anteriorly along either side of the esophagus, and was specifically not placed in a circumferential manner to avoid postoperative dysphagia as the mesh contracts over time. At 6 months, the patients in the study underwent an upper gastrointestinal (GI) barium swallow that demonstrated a decreased radiographic recurrence rate in those patients treated with the biologic mesh, from 24% in primary repair group to 9% in the biologic mesh group. The patients with radiographic recurrence were more likely to have chest pain and early satiety but did not have significantly different rates of heartburn or dysphagia according to symptom evaluation and quality of life.[6]

The same group published their long-term results at 5 years and interestingly there was no difference in recurrence rates between the simple crural closure group and the biologic mesh group at 5 years. The primary repair group had a recurrence rate of 59%, whereas the small intestine submucosa group had a recurrence rate of 54% ($P = .7$).[9] In addition, there were no statistically significant differences in frequency or severity of upper GI symptoms or in quality of life measures between the 2 groups, but there were significant improvements in symptoms and quality of life compared with the preoperative baseline.[9]

AlloMax is an alternative to porcine small intestine submucosa (SIS) and is a sterile non–cross-linked human collagen matrix that supports cellular in growth and revascularization. The group out of the University of Southern California has begun to regularly use it to reinforce their crural closure.[2] They routinely use mesh reinforcement for those with a hernia larger than 5 cm, patients with thin or atrophic crural pillars, and in all patients undergoing reoperation.[2] The group from Swedish Medical Center similarly began using AlloMax for all of their hiatal hernia repairs in 2007. Initially the mesh was placed as a posterior-only onlay reinforcement and evolved over time to a U and then to a reverse C-shaped mesh reinforcement, as there were a number of recurrences noted anteriorly and to the left of the esophagus. They had no episodes of allograft erosion into the esophagus during the study, no evidence of persistent dysphagia, and minimal difficulty with adhesions at reoperation.[25]

There is some concern for shrinkage of biologic mesh over time as the mesh is replaced with vascularized tissue and undergoes scar formation. For this reason, many investigators advocate a posterior-only[17] or a U-shaped reinforcement[8] instead of a keyhole reinforcement that is circumferential around the esophagus. As this scars over time, it may lead to increased dysphagia. With the posterior-only reinforcement, there was no increase in rates of dysphagia between those repaired with mesh and those not repaired with mesh at a follow-up of 6 months.[17]

In a meta-analysis of 22 articles dealing with biologic mesh reinforcement of hiatal hernia repairs, the 2 most commonly used mesh repairs were with SIS and human acellular cadaveric dermis (HACD). These were most commonly used in a U-shape or pantaloon fashion placed posterior to the esophagus with the limbs of the mesh encircling the esophagus. The graft could be anchored with sutures, tacks, and fibrin glue. There is level 1b data that support lower recurrence rate with biologic mesh reinforcement over the short term; however, with longer-term follow-up, there is level 2b data that this benefit is lost.[24]

AUTOLOGOUS TISSUE REINFORCEMENT

With the documented success of permanent mesh reinforcement of the hiatal repair in reducing recurrences but the ultimate increase in potentially life-threatening complications, there has been investigation into the use of autologous tissue to reinforce the hiatus during hiatal hernia repair. One potential source of this autologous tissue that has been recommended is the well-vascularized falciform ligament. In the technique described by the group from the University of Louisville, the falciform ligament is mobilized from its attachments to the anterior abdominal wall, staying as close to the abdominal wall as possible to protect the vascular supply of the pedicle flap. The flap can then be delivered beneath the left lobe of the liver and used to cover the posterior cruroplasty as an onlay mesh reinforcement.[14] The investigators report having performed this procedure on 15 patients with no significant complications or need for reintervention for the hiatal hernias.

RELAXING INCISIONS IN THE DIAPHRAGM

The radial tension created from the splaying of the crural fibers that leads to a paraesophageal hernia contributes to a significant source of hernia recurrences. The effect of tension on hernia recurrence has been well demonstrated in both inguinal and ventral abdominal hernias, leading to the practice of creating a relaxing incision to reduce some of the tension on the actual repair.[13] This incision is made in an adjacent, but less critical area of fascia or muscle, and allows the tissue in the area of interest to come together with less tension.[13] This concept when extended to the crural separation of the diaphragm would suggest that a tension-free closure of the hiatus would result in the best long-term outcomes. Bradley and colleagues[26] demonstrated that the width of the crural defect is not necessarily correlative with the degree of tension required to close the hernia; however, the shape of the defect did correlate. The oval-shaped defects had significantly higher tension then defects that were slits or tear-dropped. One mechanism to achieve this tension-free closure is to perform a relaxing incision in the right diaphragm when the crural pillars cannot be brought together without undue tension.[2] This relaxing incision is made just antero-lateral to the right crus, parallel to the inferior vena cava, and usually does not need to be more than 1 to 2 cm in length.[13] Some investigators recommend entering the ipsilateral pleural space before performing the relaxing incision to ensure that there is not any lung adhesed to the diaphragm in that area.[13] If the right crus is fibrotic or there is not adequate distance between the hiatus and the inferior vena cava, then a left-sided relaxing incision can be performed, which is created along the course of the seventh rib and not radially to avoid injury to the left-sided phrenic nerve.[2,13] The left-sided incision often must be much longer to provide adequate tension-free closure of the hiatus. The diaphragmatic defect created by the relaxing incision can then be repaired with a permanent mesh patch, such as PTFE, and the crural closure reinforced with a biologic mesh[13] Some investigators have described repairing right-sided relaxing incisions with a U-shaped biologic mesh that incorporates the reinforcement of the hiatus and the closure of the relaxing incision with a single mesh.[16] These different relaxing incisions can reduce the tension on the crural closure by approximately 50%.[26]

EXTENDED TRANSMEDIASTINAL DISSECTION

Axial tension caused by a preoperative shortened esophagus is one of the primary causes of failure of repair of paraesophageal hernias. This shortening is thought to be secondary to collagen contraction and fibrosis from exposure to gastric contents refluxing into the distal esophagus.[12] This shortening can lead to disruption of the wrap or herniation of the wrap into the mediastinum, and can lead to chest pain, dysphagia, and even strangulation.[12] Patients who are at increased risk include those with large hernias, larger than 5 cm, and those with paraesophageal hernias.[11] Horvath and colleagues[12] grouped patients with preoperative imaging concerning for a shortened esophagus into 3 groups: those with apparent short esophagus, when the esophagus was actually normal in length but appeared shortened secondary to displacement of the gastroesophageal junction, those with a truly shortened but reducible esophagus, and those with a shortened but irreducible esophagus. There is a subset of patients who have significant enough esophageal shortening that they will require an esophageal-lengthening procedure.[11] There are 5% to 8% of patients who have moderate esophageal shortening and can benefit from an extended mediastinal dissection that can effectively lengthen the esophagus such that the required 2 to 3 cm of tension-free intra-abdominal esophagus can be achieved.[11,12] In the study by Swanstrom and colleagues,[15] looking only at patients with preoperative indications placing them at higher risk for a shortened esophagus, 30% had normal-length esophagus, 50% had short esophagus that could be lengthened with mediastinal dissection alone, and 20% had significant shortening requiring a Collis gastroplasty. This supports the general conclusion that the determination of esophageal length and need for additional lengthening procedures must be made by visualization in the operating room.[12] By performing an extended mediastinal dissection, which was defined as more than 5 cm and often up to 10 cm into the mediastinum along the esophagus, in patients who had moderate esophageal shortening, it is possible to achieve comparable radiographic recurrence rates to patients with a standard-length esophagus.[11] This reserves Collis gastroplasty to only those patients in whom 2 to 3 cm of tension-free esophagus cannot be obtained after extended dissection. The avoidance of the gastroplasty decreases the potential complications of the operation, namely gastric leak and complications of ectopic gastric mucosa within the neoesophagus.[11] The addition of the extended transmediastinal dissection was able be performed without any significant added morbidity compared with the standard dissection.[11]

COLLIS GASTROPLASTY

It is a violation of one of the tenants of surgery to perform a hernia repair under tension and therefore is a similar violation to perform a fundoplication around an esophagus that is under tension. This will inherently expose the fundoplication and the hiatus to axial tension, which can lead to wrap herniation or wrap disruption.[12] When an appropriate length of intra-abdominal esophagus cannot be achieved without tension, then an esophageal-lengthening procedure is necessary to reduce axial tension.[2,4] The exact location of the gastroesophageal junction can sometimes be difficult to determine and the use of intraoperative endoscopy can be helpful in confirming that the necessary 2 to 3 cm of intra-abdominal length has been achieved.[12] The "gold standard" treatment for lengthening the esophagus is the Collis gastroplasty, which was originally described in 1963, being achieved by going through the chest[12] and was later adapted to a combined laparoscopic and thoracoscopic procedure whereby a linear stapler inserted through the chest could be applied across the gastric fundus alongside a bougie to create a lengthened esophagus.[15] With the advent of advanced laparoscopic techniques, the Nissen and the Collis procedure are performed within the abdomen. The first technique involved a circular stapling device to buttonhole the stomach and then a second firing of a longitudinal stapler fired parallel to the esophagus alongside an esophageal bougie for a length of approximately 3 cm.[27] The gastric fundus is then wrapped around the neoesophagus. This leaves a 1-cm to 2-cm portion of gastric mucosa above the newly constructed high-pressure zone in approximately half of the patients, which can lead to ongoing acid exposure in the lower esophagus and issues with esophagitis, and therefore is an indication for close clinical follow-up.[12] The creation of a gastric staple line also increases the risk of leak in comparison with a fundoplication without a gastroplasty. A large series out of Pittsburgh indicated that they used Collis gastroplasties in 63% of the patients with giant paraesophageal hernias, but 88% of the postoperative leaks occurred in patients who had undergone Collis gastroplasties.[4] The use of the Collis gastroplasty is therefore often reserved only for those patients in whom a 2-cm to 3-cm length of intra-abdominal esophagus cannot be achieved with esophageal mobilization.

SUMMARY

Laparoscopic repair of giant paraesophageal hernias, including the positive pressure insufflation of the pleural cavity that it sometimes accompanies, is well tolerated[13] and results in significant improvement in symptoms in up 90% of patients.[1,6,19] Hernia recurrence is often clinically asymptomatic.[7] There is no significant correlation between symptomatic and radiologic outcomes.[19] The vast majority of patients have excellent symptoms and quality of life metrics with or without evidence of radiologic recurrence,[4,9] and most of the

episodes of recurrence that are documented radiographically are sliding hernias. The long-term follow-up of the natural history of these asymptomatic recurrent sliding hiatal hernias has not been performed; however, some small observational studies have indicated that they do not normally increase in size or become more symptomatic over time.[8]

Permanent mesh is now a well-accepted mechanism to reduce the risk of hernia recurrence in both inguinal and ventral hernia repairs. Permanent mesh has also reliably demonstrated a reduction in the occurrence of radiographic recurrences in the repair of hiatal hernias compared with suture cruroplasty alone.[18] This decrease in radiographic recurrence rate comes at the increased risk of mesh-related complications, some of which can be catastrophic and life-threatening. These mesh-related complications have led most institutions to recommend against the regular use of permanent mesh reinforcement of hiatal hernia repairs and it has fallen out of favor.

The hernia recurrence rates following the repair of complex paraesophageal hernias have subsequently decreased through the combination of biologic mesh reinforcement and reduction of axial tension through extended mediastinal dissection and esophageal-lengthening procedures, such as the Collis gastroplasty. The Southern California group reported a radiographic hernia recurrence rate of 42% in 2000,[7] but with increased utilization of AlloMax biologic mesh and more liberal use of esophageal-lengthening procedures they reported a radiographic recurrence rate of 12% in 2011.[8] The long-term durability of reinforcement of the hiatus with a biologic mesh is still somewhat uncertain, given that the absorbable nature of this type of mesh may lead the repair to gradually weaken over time and ultimately fail with longer-term follow-up.[9] Improvements in the quality and material for biologic mesh repairs will continue to improve in the near future, and these improvements may help to address some of the current structural shortcomings.

The ideal operative solution to giant paraesophageal hernias is likely to involve a combination of the modalities discussed, with the intraoperative assessment of both esophageal length and crural closure tension being of utmost importance. The addition of surgical adjuncts, such as extended transmediastinal dissection, Collis gastroplasty, and biologic mesh reinforcement, are likely all necessary, on an individualized basis, to address these 2 primary causes of hernia recurrence.

REFERENCES

1. Swanstrom LL, Jobe BA, Kinzie LR, et al. Esophageal motility and outcomes following laparoscopic paraesophageal hernia repair and fundoplication. Am J Surg 1999;177(5):359–63.
2. Alicuben ET, Worrell SG, DeMeester SR. Impact of crural relaxing incisions, Collis gastroplasty, and non-cross-linked human dermal mesh crural reinforcement on early hiatal hernia recurrence rates. J Am Coll Surg 2014;219(5):988–92.
3. Stylopoulos N, Gazelle GS, Rattner DW. Paraesophageal hernias: operation or observation? Ann Surg 2002;236(4):492–500 [discussion: 500–91].
4. Luketich JD, Nason KS, Christie NA, et al. Outcomes after a decade of laparoscopic giant paraesophageal hernia repair. J Thorac Cardiovasc Surg 2010; 139(2):395–404, 404.e1.
5. Stylopoulos N, Rattner DW. The history of hiatal hernia surgery: from Bowditch to laparoscopy. Ann Surg 2005;241(1):185–93.
6. Oelschlager BK, Pellegrini CA, Hunter J, et al. Biologic prosthesis reduces recurrence after laparoscopic paraesophageal hernia repair: a multicenter, prospective, randomized trial. Ann Surg 2006;244(4):481–90.
7. Hashemi M, Peters JH, DeMeester TR, et al. Laparoscopic repair of large type III hiatal hernia: objective followup reveals high recurrence rate. J Am Coll Surg 2000;190(5):553–60 [discussion: 560–1].
8. Zehetner J, Demeester SR, Ayazi S, et al. Laparoscopic versus open repair of paraesophageal hernia: the second decade. J Am Coll Surg 2011;212(5):813–20.
9. Oelschlager BK, Pellegrini CA, Hunter JG, et al. Biologic prosthesis to prevent recurrence after laparoscopic paraesophageal hernia repair: long-term follow-up from a multicenter, prospective, randomized trial. J Am Coll Surg 2011;213(4):461–8.
10. Stadlhuber RJ, Sherif AE, Mittal SK, et al. Mesh complications after prosthetic reinforcement of hiatal closure: a 28-case series. Surg Endosc 2009; 23(6):1219–26.
11. O'Rourke RW, Khajanchee YS, Urbach DR, et al. Extended transmediastinal dissection: an alternative to gastroplasty for short esophagus. Arch Surg 2003;138(7):735–40.
12. Horvath KD, Swanstrom LL, Jobe BA. The short esophagus: pathophysiology, incidence, presentation, and treatment in the era of laparoscopic antireflux surgery. Ann Surg 2000;232(5):630–40.
13. Greene CL, DeMeester SR, Zehetner J, et al. Diaphragmatic relaxing incisions during laparoscopic paraesophageal hernia repair. Surg Endosc 2013; 27(12):4532–8.
14. Park AE, Hoogerboord CM, Sutton E. Use of the falciform ligament flap for closure of the esophageal hiatus in giant paraesophageal hernia. J Gastrointest Surg 2012;16(7):1417–21.
15. Swanstrom LL, Marcus DR, Galloway GQ. Laparoscopic Collis gastroplasty is the treatment of choice for the shortened esophagus. Am J Surg 1996; 171(5):477–81.
16. Auyang ED, Pellegrini CA. How I do it: laparoscopic paraesophageal hernia repair. J Gastrointest Surg 2012;16(7):1406–11.
17. Goers TA, Cassera MA, Dunst CM, et al. Paraesophageal hernia repair with biomesh does not increase postoperative dysphagia. J Gastrointest Surg 2011;15(10):1743–9.
18. Tam V, Winger DG, Nason KS. A systematic review and meta-analysis of mesh vs suture cruroplasty in laparoscopic large hiatal hernia repair. Am J Surg 2016;211(1):226–38.
19. Furnee EJ, Draaisma WA, Simmermacher RK, et al. Long-term symptomatic outcome and radiologic assessment of laparoscopic hiatal hernia repair. Am J Surg 2010;199(5):695–701.
20. Frantzides CT, Madan AK, Carlson MA, et al. A prospective, randomized trial of laparoscopic polytetrafluoroethylene (PTFE) patch repair vs simple cruroplasty for large hiatal hernia. Arch Surg 2002; 137(6):649–52.
21. Granderath FA, Schweiger UM, Kamolz T, et al. Laparoscopic Nissen fundoplication with prosthetic hiatal closure reduces postoperative intrathoracic wrap herniation: preliminary results of a prospective randomized functional and clinical study. Arch Surg 2005;140(1):40–8.
22. Muller-Stich BP, Holzinger F, Kapp T, et al. Laparoscopic hiatal hernia repair: long-term outcome with the focus on the influence of mesh reinforcement. Surg Endosc 2006;20(3):380–4.
23. Petersen LF, McChesney SL, Daly SC, et al. Permanent mesh results in long-term symptom improvement and patient satisfaction without increasing adverse outcomes in hiatal hernia repair. Am J Surg 2014;207(3):445–8 [discussion: 448].
24. Antoniou SA, Pointner R, Granderath FA, et al. The use of biological meshes in diaphragmatic defects—an evidence-based review of the literature. Front Surg 2015;2:56.
25. Bell RC, Fearon J, Freeman KD. Allograft dermal matrix hiatoplasty during laparoscopic primary fundoplication, paraesophageal hernia repair, and reoperation for failed hiatal hernia repair. Surg Endosc 2013;27(6):1997–2004.
26. Bradley DD, Louie BE, Farivar AS, et al. Assessment and reduction of diaphragmatic tension during hiatal hernia repair. Surg Endosc 2015;29(4): 796–804.
27. Johnson AB, Oddsdottir M, Hunter JG. Laparoscopic Collis gastroplasty and Nissen fundoplication. A new technique for the management of esophageal foreshortening. Surg Endosc 1998; 12(8):1055–60.

Endoluminal Therapies for Esophageal Perforations and Leaks

Jeffrey R. Watkins, MD, Alexander S. Farivar, MD*

KEYWORDS

- Endoluminal therapy • Esophageal perforation • Endoluminal clips • Esophageal stents
- Endoluminal vacuum therapy • Endoscopic vacuum therapy

KEY POINTS

- Esophageal perforation has historically been a devastating condition resulting in high morbidity and mortality.
- The use of endoluminal therapies to treat esophageal leaks and perforations has grown exponentially over the last decade and offers many advantages over traditional surgical intervention in the appropriate circumstances.
- Endoscopic clip placement may be used as first-line therapy for acute spontaneous esophageal perforations, iatrogenic perforations, anastomotic leaks, and chronic fistulas.
- Placement of covered esophageal stents has proven to be both technically and clinically successful for the indication of esophageal perforation or leak over the last decade.
- Endoluminal vacuum therapy has proven to be effective not only for salvage therapy but also for primary treatment of esophageal perforation, including spontaneous and iatrogenic perforation.

INTRODUCTION

Esophageal perforation has historically been a devastating condition resulting in high morbidity and mortality. There are many different causes of esophageal perforation, including spontaneous, iatrogenic (instrumentation or postoperative), malignancy, foreign body, or chemical corrosion. Regardless of the cause, the traditional treatment of upper gastrointestinal (GI) perforation has been either conservative management, if the injury meets specific criteria, or open surgical repair. Even in the face of prompt operative intervention, the mortality of esophageal perforation remains high. Therefore, new interventional endoscopic techniques, including endoscopic clips, covered metal stents, and endoluminal vacuum therapy (EVT), have been developed over the last several years to manage esophageal perforation and attempt to decrease the related morbidity and mortality.

The use of endoluminal therapies to treat esophageal leaks and perforations has grown exponentially over the last decade and offers many advantages compared with traditional surgical intervention in the appropriate circumstances. The need for a thoracotomy or laparotomy may be negated. Endoscopic treatment can result in an incisionless procedure if no associated drainage procedure is needed. In addition, many endoscopic therapies offer shorter hospital stays and shorter recovery times. Even with these new techniques, however, every patient with esophageal perforation must be carefully approached and the right therapy tailored to the individual. Often, a combined endoscopic and thoracoscopic

Disclosure Statement: The authors have nothing to disclose.
Division of Thoracic Surgery, Swedish Cancer Institute, 1101 Madison Street Suite 900, Seattle, WA 98104, USA
* Corresponding author.
E-mail address: alex.farivar@swedish.org

Thorac Surg Clin 28 (2018) 541–554
https://doi.org/10.1016/j.thorsurg.2018.07.002

approach may be used, thus maximizing the strength and minimizing the morbidity of each modality.

This article addresses the following key points:

- Cause, timing, and diagnosis of esophageal perforation
- Indications for management of perforation
- Endoluminal therapies
  - Endoscopic clip placement
  - Self-expanding covered metal stents
  - Endoluminal wound vacuum systems
- Outcomes of endoluminal therapy.

ESOPHAGEAL PERFORATION
Incidence and Demographics

The incidence of esophageal perforation varies within the literature and is often based on case reports from large tertiary institutions; therefore, a true population incidence is unknown in the global setting. Estimates place the incidence of age-standardized esophageal perforation at around 3.1 per 1,000,000 per year but this may vary depending on the geographic region.[1] There is a slight predominance in male patients and typical patients are in their sixties.[2]

Etiologic Factors

Esophageal perforations are often grouped together in one broad category; however, they do not come from a single cause but from several different causes. The most common cause is iatrogenic and usually occurs after endoscopic procedures.[3] Endoscopic dilation for strictures and achalasia, in particular, are associated with a high rate of perforation and even standard upper endoscopy is associated with a perforation rate of around 0.033% and carries with it significant morbidity and mortality.[4] Foregut surgery is associated with a 1% esophageal perforation rate, and suture placement during laparoscopic antireflux surgery is believed to be the most common cause.[5] Iatrogenic perforation may also be the result of inadvertent injury to the esophagus at the time of an unrelated surgery.[6–9] Postoperative leak or fistula after esophagectomy can be high as 20% but is associated with 40% of post-esophagectomy mortalities.[10,11]

Spontaneous rupture of the esophagus without clearly identified pathophysiology is often related to a sudden increase in intraabdominal pressure as a result from retching or vomiting. Commonly referred to as Boerhaave syndrome, this entity was first described in 1724 and is a result of spontaneous transmural rupture of the esophagus.[12] Other rare causes of spontaneous rupture, such as weight lifting, defecation, and blunt trauma, have been reported.[13]

Ingestion of caustic liquids is a common cause of esophageal perforation in the pediatric population. Items such as drain cleaner, batteries, or other household solutions are the main cause and can be extremely damaging to the esophagus, often leading to caustic perforation.[14] Acid ingestion can result in coagulative necrosis but is less likely to cause perforation compared with alkali solutions, which are associated with liquefactive necrosis and cause transmural perforation.[15]

Perforations in the setting of malignancy can also occur, either spontaneously or during endoscopic workup, including ultrasonic staging. For the purposes of this article, this cause is excluded because it likely requires a different management algorithm of immediate resection versus palliation, depending on several patient and oncologic factors, and a more protracted postoperative course in that setting may not be appropriate.

Location

A recent review identified 20 studies reporting on the position of perforation in the esophagus. The most common location of esophageal perforation is thoracic at 72.6%. Perforations of the cervical esophagus make up 15.2% of all perforations and abdominal location is the least frequent at 12.5%.[16]

Signs and Symptoms

The hallmark of esophageal perforation is chest pain, although this is present in only about 70% of patients with full-thickness perforation. The pain associated with perforation is often sharp, severe, acute in onset, radiates to the back or shoulder, and often follows some inciting event. Emesis and shortness of breath may also be associated. The classically described Mackler triad consists of emesis, chest pain, and subcutaneous emphysema.[17]

Cervical perforation often manifests as neck pain, although aerodigestive changes, such as dysphonia, cervical dysphagia, hoarseness, and subcutaneous emphysema, may also be present.[18] Abdominal perforation often presents as acute abdominal pain and peritonitis.

Systemic signs resulting from inflammatory response and sepsis are often delayed but early on (within 24 hours) include tachycardia and fever. If treatment is not initiated, overwhelming sepsis resulting from mediastinitis manifests as multisystem organ failure and severe sepsis, which occurs in approximately 25% of patients presenting with perforation.[16]

Diagnosis

Patients with a high clinical suspicion of esophageal perforation should be evaluated with appropriate radiographic investigations. Although no prospective studies exist, a review of 15 studies looking at diagnostic modalities in patients who were ultimately diagnosed with esophageal perforation reports that computed tomography (CT) scans resulted in 38.7% confirmed diagnoses, whereas endoscopy and oral-contrasted esophagogram resulted in a confirmed diagnosis in 37.4% and 36.6% of patients, respectively.[16] A single diagnostic modality in itself has relatively low diagnostic accuracy, although each study has its advantages and, used in conjunction with other tests, increases the diagnostic yield. A CT scan can identify masses, abscess, effusions, or other drainable collections needing additional therapy and is the preferred first-line diagnostic modality. This is usually followed by oral-contrasted esophagogram if an active leak is suspected, followed by endoscopy, which can be therapeutic in addition to diagnostic.

Timing of Intervention

Early diagnosis and intervention plays a vital role in maximizing favorable outcomes for esophageal perforation. Unfortunately, only about half of patients with perforation are seen in the hospital within the initial 24-hour window.[16] The literature is varied regarding early presentation and mortality. Several single-center studies demonstrate a significant decrease of almost 50% mortality and hospital length of stay when patients present less than 24 hours after perforation.[19,20] Other centers have shown that with aggressive management the increase in mortality and complications seen in late presentation can be ameliorated and that time to treatment is less significant.[2,21]

Open Surgical Management

Although open surgical intervention has traditionally been the standard in management of esophageal perforation, over the last decade a shift has occurred in regard to the choice of primary treatment. There is a paucity of randomized prospective trials looking at the optimal management of esophageal perforation, and even the retrospective data is inconclusive in terms of optimal management strategies.[16] Although a detailed look at surgical options is outside the scope of this discussion, it is worth examining some outcomes to better compare with an endoluminal approach.

Over the last decade, the proportion of patients with esophageal perforation managed by open surgical intervention has decreased and now comprises less than half of all cases.[16] Thoracotomy and primary 3-layer repair of the esophagus comprises much of surgical management, followed by wide local drainage alone, esophagectomy, diversion, and T-tube placement.[21] Overall mortality after open surgery for esophageal perforation is around 20%; however, prompt surgical intervention can reduce that mortality by 50% to 70%.[22]

Despite the advances and successes in endoscopic management of esophageal perforation, it must be reiterated that the surgical principle of source control must be the guiding force behind the management of leaks. The patient with extraesophageal contamination is done a disservice if the esophageal pathologic issue is managed endoscopically while mediastinal or pleural contamination is left untreated. The liberal use of open and percutaneous drainage procedures in conjunction with endoluminal therapy is a key concept in the successful management of these patients.

ENDOLUMINAL STRATEGIES
Endoscopic Clips

The idea of closing GI defects with metallic clips dates back at least to 1975, with the first clips being used for hemostasis.[23] Endoscopic clip application for postoperative anastomotic leak was first attempted in 1995.[24] Since then, the indications for endoscopic clipping have broadened to include perforation, fistula, and natural orifice transluminal endoscopic surgery (NOTES) closure, among others, and have gained prominence over the last decade.

The first endoscopic clips were deployed through the working channel of the scope. Although generally effective for many endoluminal therapies, such as hemostasis, mucosectomy closures, and smaller perforations, they are limited to smaller applications by size and closing force. Even with these limitations, they can be effective in closing lower GI perforations in 59% to 83% of cases.[25,26] These clips stay attached to the mucosa for between 2 to 4 weeks.[27] The bear-trap–like over-the-scope clip (OTSC) system (Ovesco Endoscopy AG, Tübingen, Germany) was developed and circumvents many of the limitations of the through-the-scope clips. By avoiding the working channel, the clip area is much larger and can be used on lesions up to 30 mm in the lower GI tract, with a much stronger closing force.[28,29] In addition, a through-the-scope specialized twin-grasper or anchor may be used to better approximate the affected tissue. The OTSC may reduce the surgery rate in iatrogenic perforations compared with through-the-scope clips.[30] The difference between the 2 types of clips can be seen in **Fig. 1**.

Indications

Endoscopic clip placement may be used as first-line therapy for acute spontaneous esophageal perforations, iatrogenic perforations, anastomotic leaks, and chronic fistulas. Acute perforations with minimal inflammation are associated with higher clinical success rates than chronic fistulas or leaks with inflamed edges.[31] In addition, higher success rates are associated with clip placement as a primary therapy rather than a secondary therapy after previous failure of therapy.[32] There is no size limit for successful closure, although the average lesion size of successful closure is around 8 mm with increasing rates of failure associated with lesions longer than 13 mm.[33,34]

Techniques and strategies

It is helpful to identify the esophageal lesion radiographically before implementing endoluminal therapy if the lesion has not been created and identified immediately endoscopically. This can aid the surgeon in deciding on the appropriate therapy, including clip size and location, and whether other concomitant interventions such as feeding tubes or drainage procedures are necessary. The procedure should be performed under general anesthesia and all equipment should be

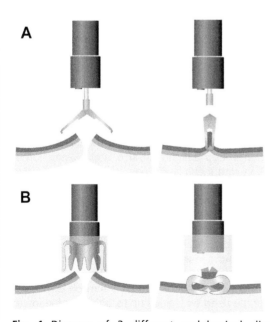

Fig. 1. Diagram of 2 different endoluminal clip deployment mechanisms. Through-the-scope clips (*A*) can be deployed through the working channel obviating withdrawal of the scope to reload, whereas OTSCs (*B*) offer greater tissue purchase and closing force.

ready in the room. An esophagoscopy should be performed to identify the lesion and any other abnormalities of the GI tract. Once the lesion is identified, the correct clip size should be chosen if the pathologic portion is appropriately sized and has reasonably healthy mucosal edges so that the clips will adhere and seal. For smaller lesions, less than a centimeter in diameter, through-the-scope clips may suffice. The clip is passed through the scope and adjusted to generously grab both edges of the lesion. Suction is applied to gather the most tissue possible and the assistant closes the jaws tight but does not fire. The clip and lesion are inspected and, if appropriately reapproximated, then fired. If the lesion requires 2 or more clips, the process is repeated until the lesion is properly closed.

If the lesion is too large or bulky, an OTSC may be used. Depending on the type of lesion, 3 different clip types are available: spiked teeth, blunt teeth, and longer pointed teeth. The pointed teeth clip is used for gastric full-thickness closure, the spiked teeth clip can be used on all tissue, and the blunt teeth clip is recommended for acute lesions with soft tissue. There are several methods to approximate the tissue to be clipped. The traditional suction method can be used in which the lesion is suctioned through the cap on the end of the scope to approximate the edges in a circumferential manner. This has been proposed as the superior method in GI lesions with thickened or edematous edges.[35] A through-the-scope single or double grasper may also be used with the purpose of bringing together the tissue edges. Once the scope and tissue are in position, the hand wheel on the scope handle is cranked and the clip is clamped and released.

The postprocedure patient should be made nil per os until a contrast esophagogram can be obtained, usually within 24 hours. Once there is no evidence of leak, the patient can start clear liquids and advance to a full-liquid or soft-mechanical diet. If there is an ongoing leak, the treating physician should consider what additional options, endoscopic or otherwise, are appropriate. This will depend on size and containment of leak, as well as clinical parameters. If the clips are unlikely to be successful during the initial consideration of application, then the authors warn against using them because the hardware may complicate subsequent intervention, be it stent or primary operative repair.

Complications

Few complications of endoscopic clip placement for perforation and leak have been reported in the literature. Most are associated with minor, self-resolving outcomes. Malfunction in clip deployment, contralateral esophageal ulceration, and tongue laceration have all been described.[35,36] There is a report of esophageal perforation associated with endoscopic perforation before clip placement that was successfully treated with surgery.[37]

Outcomes

Outcomes and results of larger studies looking at closure of esophageal perforations and leaks is shown in **Table 1**. There is a paucity of randomized prospective trials and most of the studies consist of retrospective single-center case series with a few retrospective multicenter trials. Two prospective trials enrolled 13 and 5 esophageal perforation subjects each.[37,38] In addition, most studies looking at the use of endoscopic clips include the entirety of the GI tract, which makes identifying only esophageal lesions more difficult. These low enrollment numbers highlight the difficulty in comparing outcomes in the esophageal perforation population because the condition occurs relatively infrequently and is thus difficult to study prospectively. Clinical success, which is measured by recovery from the perforation with no further surgical intervention, ranges from 56% to 100%. The authors believe that a bear-trap–like clip may be a reasonable option for an acute, immediately recognized small perforation that still maintains healthy (not inflamed) mucosal edges; however, as the time from injury and tissue inflammation increases, this may be a less effective and successful intervention. In the authors' practice, use of this intervention for perforations and leaks is limited relative to other endoluminal strategies.

Stents

The use of endoluminal stents in the treatment of esophageal perforation is not a new concept and in fact dates back to as early as the late nineteenth century.[39] The first tubes consisted of ivory and silver but gradually evolved over the next decades to include plastic and polyethylene. These tubes were difficult to place and problems with migration limited their use. Their modern incarnation, the self-expanding metal stent (SEMS) were introduced in the 1990s and borrow from endovascular stent designs. These stents are presented in a compact format easily introduced into the esophagus and expand to a fixed diameter. Synthetic wall coverings made from silicone, polyurethane, or other polymers were added to decrease the rate of extraction complications and fistulae.

Indications

The indications for using a SEMS have broadened over the course of their development and, with improving technology, their use has expanded. Because of the limitations of early metal stents and the high incidence of erosion, their use was limited to palliative procedures for malignant stricture and tracheoesophageal fistula.[40] The first

Table 1
Review of outcomes of endoscopic clip placement

Author, Year	Study Type	Subjects (n)	Success	Indications	Notes
Lee, et al,[38] 2017	Prospective	13	74%	A, I, F	No major complications
Otsuka, et al,[66] 2017	Retrospective	3	100%	S	1 prolonged hospitalization
Kobara, et al,[67] 2017	Retrospective	3	85%	I	
Nasa, et al,[68] 2016	Retrospective	4	100%	F	Complication: tracheoesophageal fistula
Wedi, et al,[36] 2016	Retrospective	6	89%	I, F, S	Less success with chronic
Winder, et al,[69] 2016	Retrospective	3	82%	I, F	No major complications
Haito-Chavez, et al,[32] 2014	Review	188	60.20%	A, I, F	Primary therapy more successful
Nishiyama, et al,[70] 2013	Retrospective	14	82.60%	S, F	2 complications
Mennigen, et al,[71] 2013	Retrospective	6	79%	A	Less success with fistula
Disibeyaz, et al,[31] 2012	Retrospective	6	56%	A, I, S	Less success with fistula
Voermans, et al,[37] 2012	Prospective	5	92%	A, S	
Baron, et al,[72] 2012	Retrospective	15	65%	A, F, I	

Abbreviations: A, anastomotic leak; F, fistula; I, iatrogenic perforation; S, spontaneous perforation.

description of the use of stents in a nonpalliative setting was of a successful stent placement for treatment of iatrogenic esophageal perforation.[41] Many of the early applications of stent placement for esophageal perforation came about because of patient instability or poor candidacy for surgical intervention.[42] Successful outcomes in these patients led to broader adoption and more widespread use. Additional early stent studies examined the successful management of postesophagectomy anastomotic leak (**Fig. 2**).[43] Additional indications for stent placement include spontaneous perforation, fistulae, and iatrogenic perforation. In addition to stent placement, mediastinal or pleural drainage procedures are often required due to contamination, and nutrition should be optimized with enteral feeding tube placement. Predictors of successful clinical outcomes are linked to shorter diagnosis time and smaller luminal opening size.[44–46]

Techniques and strategies

Thorough preprocedural planning is essential for successful stent placement and optimizing patient outcomes. Reviewing patient imaging before placing the stent, whether by contrast esophagogram or CT scan, will assist in locating the source of the lesion and ensure that the right equipment is available. A CT scan also facilitates the decision of whether a concomitant drainage procedure is needed while under anesthesia (eg, thoracoscopy, tube thoracostomy).

General anesthesia should be used and fluoroscopy available in the room. Before placing the stent, esophagoscopy may better localize and assess the extent of the lesion, identify anatomic landmarks, and identify any other GI abnormalities if the problem is heretofore unknown. A careful assessment of landing zones for the stent should be considered (both in planning and endoscopically), as well as what is believed to be the appropriate diameter and length of stent.

Once the pathologic condition has been identified, landmarks are marked under fluoroscopy using radio-opaque markers, and should delineate the proximal and distal extent of the planned stent placement (some surgeons may prefer to mark the location of the lesion). A guidewire is placed under direct visualization either in the distal stomach or duodenum, facilitating deployment under fluoroscopic guidance. Choosing the correct stent can be difficult and should be based on the individual patient and the anatomy involved, including esophageal or conduit diameter. It has been advocated to somewhat oversize rather than undersize the stent to maximize the ability to seal a leak while attempting to mitigate the possibility of stent migration and maximize overlap.[47,48] Placement should be centered on the lesion itself but crossing the upper esophageal sphincter (discomfort, cough) or lower esophageal sphincter (migration, reflux) should be avoided. Placing overlapping stents usually is not necessary if proper stent placement and location is achieved but may be used or needed at the discretion of the treating physician. If the stent is placed too low, it may be grasped and adjusted proximally using the endoscope. If it is placed too proximal, pushing it distal may prove difficult and the stent may need to be replaced. If the stent does not appear to have achieved full radial deployment, a balloon dilation may be attempted with the understanding that full deployment may take up to 24 hours. Sometimes the stent will need to be sized smaller if it is too large and the edges are rolled onto itself. Several techniques have been studied to help prevent stent migration, including endoscopic suturing and clipping with favorable results.[49,50] It may be advantageous to endoscopically visualize placement of a nasogastric tube (NGT) and ensure it is traveling through and not around the stent. Fluoroscopy can help visualize the tip of the NGT in the stomach if one does not want to endoscopically pass through the stent once deployed. Other

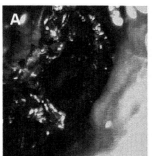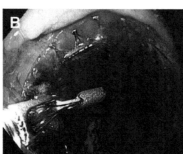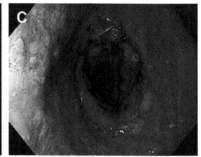

Fig. 2. Endoscopic views of esophagogastric anastomotic leak before therapy (*A*), with covered metal stent in situ (*B*) and stent therapy (*C*).

factors to consider before leaving the operating room is whether one believes an adequate distal and proximal seal have been achieved and if the distal stent allows adequate forward egress of saliva into the stomach (ie, the distal stent is not deployed against the esophageal wall such that the stent lumen has a distal obstruction). Additionally, a percutaneous endoscopic gastric tube or percutaneous gastrojejunostomy tube may be inserted before stent deployment.

After placement of a stent, a postprocedure 2-view chest radiograph establishes a baseline for stent position and can aid in identification of stent migration. The patient should be placed on nil per os and started on proton pump inhibitor therapy until a formal contrast esophagogram can be performed to assess for appropriate control or ongoing leakage. The patient may begin a soft-mechanical diet or other feeding via enteral access as deemed appropriate. There is no definitive method to determine when a stent should be removed but several studies suggest that earlier stent removal between 2 to 4 weeks is associated with better outcomes than stents left in place longer.[47,51,52]

Complications

As with every medical intervention, endoluminal stent placement is not without its risks and complications, although major complications are rare. Most of the volume of data related to stent placement and complications come from esophageal cancer studies often used for palliation or anastomotic leak. Of the complications seen, stent migration is the most common with around 20% incidence and up to 62% of stents undergo migration after anastomotic leak.[53] Other complications include tissue overgrowth, erosions or ulcers, bleeding, aspiration pneumonia, perforation, fistula, and reflux.[54] An important factor to be sorted is whether the stent is adequately sealing the leak, and both radiographic or fluoroscopic and clinical indicators will help answer that question.

Outcomes

Placement of esophageal stents has proven to be both technically and clinically successful for the indication of esophageal perforation or leak over the last decade. Several recent studies are shown in **Table 2**. There are no randomized prospective trials given the nature of the disease process; however, there are multiple retrospective multicenter and single-center case series that show clinical effectiveness ranging from 63% to 89%. Clinical success is defined as closure of the leak or perforation without the need for further intervention. The most common complication is stent migration, which occurs in 8.8% to 40% of stent placements. Mortality in these series rages from 0% to 17%. Although there is a paucity of direct comparison of closure methods, a literature review found

Table 2
Review of outcomes of endoscopic stent placement

Author, Year	Type	Subjects (n)	Success	Indication	Notes
Gonzalez, et al,[10] 2016	Retrospective	35	69%	A	18% migration, 17% mortality
Suzuki, et al,[73] 2016	Retrospective	36	85%	A, S, F	40% migration
Persson, et al,[74] 2016	Retrospective	46	63%	A	Predictors of failure: decreased preoperative performance, leakage, tracheoesophageal fistula
Van Halsema, et al,[75] 2015	Review	643	77%	A, I, S, F	17% migration, 10% mortality
Ben-David, et al,[76] 2014	Retrospective	76	89%	I, S	>30% prolonged intubation
Freeman, et al,[51] 2014	Retrospective	29	86%	A	17% migration, 0% mortality
Gubler, et al,[77] 2014	Retrospective	113	79%	I, S, F	9% migration, 9% mortality
Orive-Calzada, et al,[78] 2014	Retrospective	56	79%	I, S, F	20% migration, 16% mortality
Persson, et al,[46] 2014	Retrospective	40	83%	I, S, F	No stent-related complications
El Hajj, et al,[45] 2014	Retrospective	54	83%	A, I, S, F	28% migration

successful closure was achieved by placement of clips and stents in almost equal numbers but limited by a small stent cohort.[55] Compared with open repair, stent placement for acute esophageal perforation was associated with decreased morbidity (4% vs 43%, $P = .02$), length of stay, time to oral intake, and cost.[51]

Endoluminal Vacuum Therapy

Within the last decade, EVT has emerged as an effective technique in the endoluminal treatment of esophageal perforation and leak. Originally described in 2003 for the endoluminal treatment of rectal anastomotic leaks, the technique was adapted for use in the upper GI tract later in the decade.[56,57]

EVT is known in the literature by several different names: endoscopic vacuum therapy, endoscopic vacuum-assisted closure, and Endo-sponge (B. Braun Melsungen AG, Melsungen, Germany) therapy. Regardless of the name, the therapy uses the same principles as cutaneous negative-therapy vacuum-assisted devices. A porous wound sponge attached to a NGT is placed either intraluminal or in the abscess cavity under endoscopic guidance and negative pressure is applied (**Fig. 3**). This results in decreased edema, removal of infected secretions, and gradual closure of the lesion. The only currently available commercial device, the Endo-Sponge, is approved by the US Food and Drug Administration only for treatment of rectal anastomotic leaks. Because of this limitation, the commonly available Wound V.A.C. (Lifecell, Bridgewater, NJ, USA) is often adapted for use in EVT.

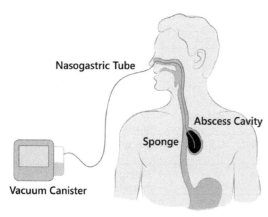

Nasogastric Tube

Abscess Cavity

Sponge

Vacuum Canister

Fig. 3. Diagram of the basic endoluminal vacuum setup. A black wound sponge is attached to the end of a 14F NGT and placed endoscopically into the abscess cavity or luminal defect. The NGT is then attached to a negative pressure wound vacuum therapy system.

Indications

The initial uses for EVT described in the literature were for patients with postsurgical anastomotic leaks, poor surgical candidates, or patients who had failed other therapies.[57,58] Although endoscopic clip and stent placement have been shown effective in small to moderate-sized acute perforation or leaks, they have been proven less so with chronic fistulae or other larger defects. EVT therapy is limited only by the size of the sponge used and can be placed intraluminal or intracavitary. The therapy has even proven successful in a complete circumferential postesophagectomy anastomotic breakdown, sparing the patient a cervical esophagostomy (**Fig. 4**).[59] It can also be used as a bridge therapy in the postesophagectomy conduit to tracheal fistula, allowing control of gastric fluid and allowing the soiled lungs to heal before formal repair. It is an ideal therapy for anastomotic leaks in that mediastinal soilage can be addressed from the intraluminal source of the leak and, in select circumstances, without having to make a percutaneous incision.

Recent studies have shown the EVT therapy to be effective not only for salvage therapy but also for primary treatment of esophageal perforation, including spontaneous and iatrogenic perforation. In addition, the technique has found a place in the management of bariatric surgery complications.[60] A emerging technique is using percutaneous drains for a rendezvous procedure in which difficult-to-reach areas can be accessed with promising results.[61,62]

Techniques and strategies

As with other endoluminal therapies, extensive preprocedural preparation is key to obtaining successful clinical outcomes. Preoperative imaging, such as contrast esophagogram or CT scan, is helpful in assessing the extent of the lesion, as well as the location. The procedure should be performed under general anesthesia in either the endoscopic suite or the operating room. Esophagoscopy is helpful in identifying the lesion and is necessary to determine the size and extent of the cavity to properly measure the sponge. Thought should be given to placing an enteral feeding tube at the time of initial therapy because placing a nasoduodenal feeding tube beside the NGT is cumbersome and contributes to even more patient discomfort.

Once the lesion has been identified and sized, the sponge apparatus must be prepared. A topical wound vacuum therapy kit may be used and the appropriate size chosen, usually small or medium. The black polyurethane sponge is trimmed to size using scissors in a shape that will fill the defect,

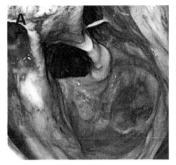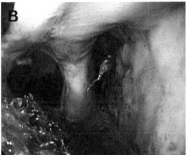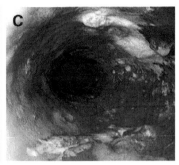

Fig. 4. Complete disruption of cervical esophagogastric anastomosis and mediastinal abscess (*A*) with application of EVT (*B*). Complete resolution after 2 months of endoscopic intervention (*C*).

remembering that the sponge system will be placed straight in, rather than on its side (**Fig. 5**). Once the sponge is cut to size, a 14F NGT is placed through the nares and out the mouth. This is performed before the sponge is placed; otherwise the sponge cannot pass through the nose. Once the tube is out of the mouth, it is trimmed so that the sponge can cover all the distal NGT holes with approximately a centimeter of excess sponge at the end. This is accomplished by creating a hole in the sponge with the scissors and passing the trimmed NGT into the hole so that the holes are covered, including the trimmed end hole. This is then sutured into place by passing a permanent suture attached to a straight needle through the proximal sponge, tube, out the other side through sponge, and back again through all 3, creating a mattress suture. This is repeated at the distal end while leaving a 2 to 3 cm loop as a handle for the grasper. The proximal end of the NGT is attached to the vacuum canister at minus 125 to 175 mm Hg after the sponge is placed in its appropriate endoluminal position.

The suture loop at the end of the tube or sponge is grasped with the endoscopic grasper and the endoscope is passed into the mouth and esophagus with the sponge trailing. Sometimes it is necessary to manually help the sponge pass through the oropharynx. Once the sponge has passed into the esophagus, it is dragged past the defect, then pulled proximally into place. It is easier to pull the sponge into place than to push it forward. When in the cavity, the sponge position can be finely adjusted using the endoscope. Once in place, the suction is started, and the sponge will adhere to the lumen walls, fixing into place. An endoluminal stent may be used in the esophagus to secure the sponge into place, although this is usually unnecessary with large abscess cavities. For larger complete anastomotic dehiscence, a stent may help maintain luminal continuity and secure the sponge into place outside the stent.

Proper timing for changing of the sponge is not absolute and must be decided based on the individual patient. Defects with large cavities, sepsis, or an increased burden of purulence may be changed earlier. It is common to wait 3 to 5 days between therapies, although there is no good evidence to support shorter or longer times periods. Procalcitonin serum levels have been used to help guide the duration of sponge therapy between changes.[58] During the procedure, if the sponge is difficult to extract from the wall, the sponge may be soaked with water to more easily

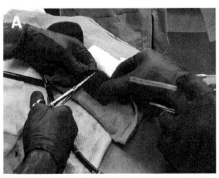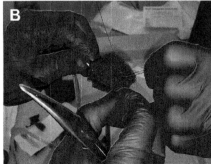

Fig. 5. Preparing the sponge in the operating room by trimming it to size (*A*) and securing it to the end of an NGT after placing it through the nares (*B*).

remove it from the surrounding tissue. The replacement of the sponge with a newly created sponge and NGT then proceeds as previously described. After several procedures, the defect will shrink in size and develop healthy granulation tissue. The endpoint of therapy should be the appearance of healthy tissue or shrinkage of the defect to the point at which a sponge no longer fits in the lesion. At this point, the sponge may be replaced by a stent alone.

Once therapy has been discontinued, a contrast esophagogram can be obtained within 24 hours to identify any free perforations or other abnormalities, although after several sponge changes one is unlikely to find a freely leaking perforation. Obtaining an esophagogram, placing a stent, feeding a patient by mouth, and discharging a patient are then done at the discretion of the treating physician.

Complications

Endoluminal wound vacuum therapy is generally well-tolerated with little of the morbidity and mortality associated with esophageal perforation. The most common complication is stricture requiring dilation because the granulation tissue forming in the likely ischemic bed can be vigorous. Other complications include hemorrhage, nasal trauma, prolonged sepsis, and death, although major complications occur in less than 10% of patients. This is also a high-maintenance, anesthesia-intensive, and resource-intensive option because there are frequent returns to the operating room. This must be balanced against the benefits and risks of diversion that would typically be done in some of these more extensive anastomotic dehiscences.

Outcomes

Recent literature shows favorable outcomes in regard to clinical success of endoluminal wound vacuum therapy (**Table 3**). There are no randomized trials but the largest prospective trial to date includes 52 subjects with spontaneous, iatrogenic, and postoperative esophageal perforation, with 94% clinical success rate but complicated by 2 mortalities associated with procedural hemorrhage, in addition to 4 strictures.[63] The largest retrospective review to date identified a mortality rate of 12.8% in 179 subjects.[64] This is concordant with another retrospective case series comparing surgery, stent placement, and vacuum therapy in which the mortality was 50%, 83%, and 12%, respectively.[65] One of the drawbacks of this therapy is the length of treatment and the number of interventions required for clinical success. Average length of therapy ranged from 12 to 36 days, with and average number

Table 3
Review of outcomes of endoluminal vacuum therapy

Author, Year	Type	Subjects (n)	Success	Length of Therapy	Average Changes	Indications	Notes
Laukoetter, et al,[79] 2017	Prospective	52	94.2%	22 d	6	A, I, S	4 strictures, 2 mortalities: hemorrhage
Newton, et al,[64] 2016	Review	179	91%	NA	NA	NA	Overall mortality 12.8%
Leeds, et al,[80] 2016	Retrospective	6	100%	35.8 d	7.2	I	No major complications
Heits, et al,[81] 2014	Retrospective	10	90%	19 d	5.4	I, F, S	1 mortality, 1 reoperation
Bludau, et al,[82] 2014	Retrospective	14	86%	12.1 d	3.9	A, I, S	2 mortalities: sepsis
Schniewind, et al,[65] 2013	Retrospective	17	83%	NA	NA	A	Mortality 12% in sponge group, 50% in surgery, 83% in stent
Wedemeyer, et al,[83] 2010	Prospective	10	88%	23 d	7	A	No major complications
Ahrens, et al,[84] 2010	Prospective	5	100%	28 d	9	A	2 dilations resulting in 1 mortality

Abbreviation: NA, not applicable.

of interventions from 4 to 9 sponge changes. Even though this is still an emerging technology, early results show a reduced morbidity and mortality compared with other therapies, and an excellent clinical success rate. In the authors' opinion, outcomes with perforation are superior to that of fistulae.

SUMMARY

In practice, the use of endoluminal therapies for esophageal perforation or leak is based on the individual patient's pathologic issue and the familiarity of the surgeon with the aforementioned techniques. Endoscopic clip placement is rarely used in the authors' practice except in very specific cases of early acute perforation with minimal inflammation, smaller size (<5 mm), and absence of chronic fistula. The presence of inflammation, poor tissue quality, larger size, and indurated wound edges precludes the use of endoscopic clips. In these patients, a SEMS has proven to be more appropriate and is placed with minimal complications and often excellent results. In cases of larger anastomotic break-down, local contamination, chronic fistula, or large abscess cavity, however, EVT has proven successful in cases in which other endoluminal modalities would be inadequate.

Esophageal perforation is an uncommon but morbid entity with many different causes. The traditional standard treatment involved open surgical intervention with drainage and repair or diversion. Recent technological advances have allowed endoluminal therapies to become more widely adopted. Interventions such as clipping, stenting, and EVT have been shown to be as effective as open surgical management of esophageal leak in the appropriate circumstances. In addition, novel endoluminal therapies can minimize morbidity and mortality compared with traditional therapy, and may even spare patients from being diverted. It is important that the esophageal surgeon become familiar with these new techniques to expand their armamentarium in treating patients with esophageal perforation or leaks.

REFERENCES

1. Vidarsdottir H, Blondal S, Alfredsson H, et al. Oesophageal perforations in Iceland: a whole population study on incidence, aetiology and surgical outcome. Thorac Cardiovasc Surg 2010;58(8):476–80.
2. Bhatia P, Fortin D, Inculet RI, et al. Current concepts in the management of esophageal perforations: a twenty-seven year Canadian experience. Ann Thorac Surg 2011;92(1):209–15.
3. Vallböhmer D, Hölscher AH, Hölscher M, et al. Options in the management of esophageal perforation: analysis over a 12-year period. Dis Esophagus 2010;23(3):185–90.
4. Merchea A, Cullinane DC, Sawyer MD, et al. Esophagogastroduodenoscopy-associated gastrointestinal perforations: a single-center experience. Surgery 2010;148(4):876–82.
5. Zhang LP, Chang R, Matthews BD, et al. Incidence, mechanisms, and outcomes of esophageal and gastric perforation during laparoscopic foregut surgery: a retrospective review of 1,223 foregut cases. Surg Endosc 2014;28(1):85–90.
6. Ahn S-H, Lee S-H, Kim ES, et al. Successful repair of esophageal perforation after anterior cervical fusion for cervical spine fracture. J Clin Neurosci 2011;18(10):1374–80.
7. Sreedharan L, Lakshmanan P, Shenfine J, et al. Thoracic vertebral osteomyelitis secondary to chronic esophageal perforation. Spine J 2009;9(4):e1–5.
8. Ozer MT, Demirbas S, Harlak A, et al. A rare complication after thyroidectomy: perforation of the oesophagus: a case report. Acta Chir Belg 2009;109(4):527–30.
9. Nérot C, Jeanneret B, Lardenois T, et al. Esophageal perforation after fracture of the cervical spine: case report and review of the literature. J Spinal Disord Tech 2002;15(6):513–8.
10. Gonzalez J-M, Servajean C, Aider B, et al. Efficacy of the endoscopic management of postoperative fistulas of leakages after esophageal surgery for cancer: a retrospective series. Surg Endosc 2016;30(11):4895–903.
11. Alanezi K, Urschel JD. Mortality secondary to esophageal anastomotic leak. Ann Thorac Cardiovasc Surg 2004;10(2):71–5.
12. Wolfson D, Barkin JS. Treatment of Boerhaave's syndrome. Curr Treat Options Gastroenterol 2007;10(1):71–7.
13. Strauss DC, Tandon R, Mason RC. Distal thoracic oesophageal perforation secondary to blunt trauma: case report. World J Emerg Surg 2007;2(1):8.
14. Rauber-Lüthy C, Kupferschmidt H. Household chemicals: management of intoxication and antidotes. EXS 2010;100:339–63.
15. Riffat F, Cheng A. Pediatric caustic ingestion: 50 consecutive cases and a review of the literature. Dis Esophagus 2009;22(1):89–94.
16. Sdralis EIK, Petousis S, Rashid F, et al. Epidemiology, diagnosis, and management of esophageal perforations: systematic review. Dis Esophagus 2017;30(8):1–6.
17. Mackler SA. Spontaneous rupture of the esophagus; an experimental and clinical study. Surg Gynecol Obstet 1952;95(3):345–56.
18. Søreide JA, Viste A. Esophageal perforation: diagnostic work-up and clinical decision-making in the

first 24 hours. Scand J Trauma Resusc Emerg Med 2011;19:66.

19. Onat S, Ulku R, Cigdem KM, et al. Factors affecting the outcome of surgically treated non-iatrogenic traumatic cervical esophageal perforation: 28 years experience at a single center. J Cardiothorac Surg 2010;5(1):46.

20. Amudhan A, Rajendran S, Raj VV, et al. Management of esophageal perforation: experience from a tertiary center in India. Dig Surg 2009;26(4):322–8.

21. Keeling WB, Miller DL, Lam GT, et al. Low mortality after treatment for esophageal perforation: a single-center experience. Ann Thorac Surg 2010; 90(5):1669–73.

22. Brinster CJ, Singhal S, Lee L, et al. Evolving options in the management of esophageal perforation. Ann Thorac Surg 2004;77(4):1475–83.

23. Hayashi I, Yonezawa TM, Kuwabara TKI. The study on staunch clip for the treatment by endoscopy. Gastrointest Endosc 1975;17:92–101.

24. Rodella L, Laterza E, De Manzoni G, et al. Endoscopic clipping of anastomotic leakages in esophagogastric surgery. Endoscopy 1998;30(5): 453–6.

25. Cho SB, Lee WS, Joo YE, et al. Therapeutic options for iatrogenic colon perforation: feasibility of endoscopic clip closure and predictors of the need for early surgery. Surg Endosc 2012;26(2):473–9.

26. Magdeburg R, Collet P, Post S, et al. Endoclipping of iatrogenic colonic perforation to avoid surgery. Surg Endosc 2008;22(6):1500–4.

27. Jensen DM, Machicado GA, Hirabayashi K. Randomized controlled study of 3 different types of hemoclips for hemostasis of bleeding canine acute gastric ulcers. Gastrointest Endosc 2006;64(5): 768–73.

28. Gubler C, Bauerfeind P. Endoscopic closure of iatrogenic gastrointestinal tract perforations with the over-the-scope clip. Digestion 2012;85(4):302–7.

29. Schurr M, Hartmann C, Ho C-N, et al. An over-the-scope clip (OTSC) system for closure of iatrogenic colon perforations: results of an experimental survival study in pigs. Endoscopy 2008;40(7):584–8.

30. Khater S, Rahmi G, Perrod G, et al. Over-the-scope clip (OTSC) reduces surgery rate in the management of iatrogenic gastrointestinal perforations. Endosc Int Open 2017;5(5):E389–94.

31. Dişibeyaz S, Köksal AŞ, Parlak E, et al. Endoscopic closure of gastrointestinal defects with an over-the-scope clip device. A case series and review of the literature. Clin Res Hepatol Gastroenterol 2012; 36(6):614–21.

32. Haito-Chavez Y, Law JK, Kratt T, et al. International multicenter experience with an over-the-scope clipping device for endoscopic management of GI defects (with video). Gastrointest Endosc 2014;80(4): 610–22.

33. Sulz MC, Bertolini R, Frei R, et al. Multipurpose use of the over-the-scope-clip system ("Bear claw") in the gastrointestinal tract: Swiss experience in a tertiary center. World J Gastroenterol 2014;20(43): 16287–92.

34. Hagel AF, Naegel A, Lindner AS, et al. Over-the-scope clip application yields a high rate of closure in gastrointestinal perforations and may reduce emergency surgery. J Gastrointest Surg 2012; 16(11):2132–8.

35. Donatelli G, Cereatti F, Dhumane P, et al. Closure of gastrointestinal defects with Ovesco clip: long-term results and clinical implications. Therap Adv Gastroenterol 2016;9(5):713–21.

36. Wedi E, Gonzalez S, Menke D, et al. One hundred and one over-the-scope-clip applications for severe gastrointestinal bleeding, leaks and fistulas. World J Gastroenterol 2016;22(5):1844–53.

37. Voermans RP, Le Moine O, von Renteln D, et al. Efficacy of endoscopic closure of acute perforations of the gastrointestinal tract. Clin Gastroenterol Hepatol 2012;10(6):603–8.

38. Lee HL, Cho JY, Cho J-H, et al. Efficacy of the over-the-scope clip system for treatment of gastrointestinal fistulas, leaks, and perforations: a korean multi-center study. Clin Endosc 2018;51(1):61–5.

39. Symonds CJ. The treatment of malignant stricture of the oesophagus by tubage or permanent catheterism. Br Med J 1887;1(1373):870–3.

40. Ell C, Hochberger J, May A, et al. Coated and uncoated self-expanding metal stents for malignant stenosis in the upper GI tract: preliminary clinical experiences with Wallstents. Am J Gastroenterol 1994; 89(9):1496–500.

41. Segalin A, Bonavina L, Lazzerini M, et al. Endoscopic management of inveterate esophageal perforations and leaks. Surg Endosc 1996;10(9): 928–32.

42. Freeman RK, Ascioti AJ, Wozniak TC. Postoperative esophageal leak management with the Polyflex esophageal stent. J Thorac Cardiovasc Surg 2007; 133(2):333–8.

43. Roy-Choudhury SH, Nicholson AA, Wedgwood KR, et al. Symptomatic malignant gastroesophageal anastomotic leak: management with covered metallic esophageal stents. AJR Am J Roentgenol 2001;176(1):161–5.

44. van Halsema E, Kappelle W, Weusten B, et al. Stent placement for benign esophageal leaks, perforations, and fistulae: a clinical prediction rule for successful leakage control. Endoscopy 2018;50(2):98–108.

45. El Hajj II, Imperiale TF, Rex DK, et al. Treatment of esophageal leaks, fistulae, and perforations with temporary stents: evaluation of efficacy, adverse events, and factors associated with successful outcomes. Gastrointest Endosc 2014;79(4):589–98.

46. Persson S, Elbe P, Rouvelas I, et al. Predictors for failure of stent treatment for benign esophageal perforations - a single center 10-year experience. World J Gastroenterol 2014;20(30):10613–9.

47. Ong GKB, Freeman RK. Endoscopic management of esophageal leaks. J Thorac Dis 2017;9(Suppl 2):S135–45.

48. van den Berg MW, Kerbert AC, van Soest EJ, et al. Safety and efficacy of a fully covered large-diameter self-expanding metal stent for the treatment of upper gastrointestinal perforations, anastomotic leaks, and fistula. Dis Esophagus 2016; 29(6):572–9.

49. Wright A, Chang A, Bedi AO, et al. Endoscopic suture fixation is associated with reduced migration of esophageal fully covered self-expandable metal stents (FCSEMS). Surg Endosc 2017;31(9): 3489–94.

50. Law R, Prabhu A, Fujii-Lau L, et al. Stent migration following endoscopic suture fixation of esophageal self-expandable metal stents: a systematic review and meta-analysis. Surg Endosc 2018; 32(2):675–81.

51. Freeman RK, Ascioti AJ, Dake M, et al. An analysis of esophageal stent placement for persistent leak after the operative repair of intrathoracic esophageal perforations. Ann Thorac Surg 2014; 97(5):1715–20.

52. Wilson JL, Louie BE, Farivar AS, et al. Fully covered self-expanding metal stents are effective for benign esophagogastric disruptions and strictures. J Gastrointest Surg 2013;17(12):2045–50.

53. Speer E, Dunst CM, Shada A, et al. Covered stents in cervical anastomoses following esophagectomy. Surg Endosc 2016;30(8):3297–303.

54. Turkyilmaz A, Eroglu A, Aydin Y, et al. Complications of metallic stent placement in malignant esophageal stricture and their management. Surg Laparosc Endosc Percutan Tech 2010;20(1):10–5.

55. Verlaan T, Voermans RP, van Berge Henegouwen MI, et al. Endoscopic closure of acute perforations of the GI tract: a systematic review of the literature. Gastrointest Endosc 2015;82(4):618–28.e5.

56. Weidenhagen R, Gruetzner K, Weilbach C, et al. Endoscopic vacuum assisted closure of anastomotic leakage after anterior resection of the rectum - a new method. Surg Endosc 2003;17(1):S92.

57. Wedemeyer J, Schneider A, Manns MP, et al. Endoscopic vacuum-assisted closure of upper intestinal anastomotic leaks. Gastrointest Endosc 2008; 67(4):708–11.

58. Smallwood NR, Fleshman JW, Leeds SG, et al. The use of endoluminal vacuum (E-Vac) therapy in the management of upper gastrointestinal leaks and perforations. Surg Endosc 2016;30(6):2473–80.

59. Watkins JR, Farivar AS, Vallieres E, et al. Successful management of complete esophagogastric anastomotic disruption using combined endoluminal vacuum therapy. Gastroenterology 2017; 152(5):S1223.

60. Leeds SG, Burdick JS. Management of gastric leaks after sleeve gastrectomy with endoluminal vacuum (E-Vac) therapy. Surg Obes Relat Dis 2016;12(7): 1278–85.

61. Pines G, Bar I, Elami A, et al. Modified endoscopic vacuum therapy for nonhealing esophageal anastomotic leak: technique description and review of literature. J Laparoendosc Adv Surg Tech A 2018;28(1): 33–40.

62. Krajinovic K, Reimer S, Kudlich T, et al. "Rendezvous technique" for intraluminal vacuum therapy of anastomotic leakage of the jejunum. Surg Case Rep 2016;2(1):114.

63. Laukoetter MG, Mennigen R, Neumann PA, et al. Successful closure of defects in the upper gastrointestinal tract by endoscopic vacuum therapy (EVT): a prospective cohort study. Surg Endosc 2017; 31(6):2687–96.

64. Newton NJ, Sharrock A, Rickard R, et al. Systematic review of the use of endo-luminal topical negative pressure in oesophageal leaks and perforations. Dis Esophagus 2016;30(3):1–5.

65. Schniewind B, Schafmayer C, Voehrs G, et al. Endoscopic endoluminal vacuum therapy is superior to other regimens in managing anastomotic leakage after esophagectomy: a comparative retrospective study. Surg Endosc 2013;27(10):3883–90.

66. Otsuka K, Murakami M, Ariyoshi T, et al. Endoscopic clipping of spontaneous esophageal rupture: case reports of three patients. Int J Surg Case Rep 2017;38:18–22.

67. Kobara H, Mori H, Fujihara S, et al. Outcomes of gastrointestinal defect closure with an over-the-scope clip system in a multicenter experience: an analysis of a successful suction method. World J Gastroenterol 2017;23(9):1645.

68. Nasa M, Sharma ZD, Choudhary NS, et al. Over-the-scope clip placement for closure of gastrointestinal fistula, postoperative leaks and refractory gastrointestinal bleed. Indian J Gastroenterol 2016;35(5): 361–5.

69. Winder JS, Kulaylat AN, Schubart JR, et al. Management of non-acute gastrointestinal defects using the over-the-scope clips (OTSCs): a retrospective single-institution experience. Surg Endosc 2016; 30(6):2251–8.

70. Nishiyama N, Mori H, Kobara H, et al. Efficacy and safety of over-the-scope clip: Including complications after endoscopic submucosal dissection. World J Gastroenterol 2013;19(18): 2752–60.

71. Mennigen R, Colombo-Benkmann M, Senninger N, et al. Endoscopic closure of postoperative gastrointestinal leakages and fistulas with the

over-the-scope clip (OTSC). J Gastrointest Surg 2013;17(6):1058–65.

72. Baron TH, Wong Kee Song LM, Ross A, et al. Use of an over-the-scope clipping device: multicenter retrospective results of the first U.S. experience (with videos). Gastrointest Endosc 2012;76(1):202–8.

73. Suzuki T, Siddiqui A, Taylor LJ, et al. Clinical outcomes, efficacy, and adverse events in patients undergoing esophageal stent placement for benign indications: a large multicenter study. J Clin Gastroenterol 2016;50(5):373–8.

74. Persson S, Rouvelas I, Kumagai K, et al. Treatment of esophageal anastomotic leakage with self-expanding metal stents: analysis of risk factors for treatment failure. Endosc Int Open 2016;4(4):E420–6.

75. Van Halsema EE, Van JE, Emo H, et al. Clinical outcomes of self-expandable stent placement for benign esophageal diseases: a pooled analysis of the literature. World J Gastrointest Endosc 2015; 16(72):135–53.

76. Ben-David K, Behrns K, Hochwald S, et al. Esophageal perforation management using a multidisciplinary minimally invasive treatment algorithm. J Am Coll Surg 2014;218(4):768–74.

77. Gubler C, Bauerfeind P. Self-expandable stents for benign esophageal leakages and perforations: long-term single-center experience. Scand J Gastroenterol 2014;49(1):23–9.

78. Orive-Calzada A, Calderón-García Á, Bernal-Martínez A, et al. Closure of benign leaks, perforations, and fistulas with temporary placement of fully covered metal stents: a retrospective analysis. Surg Laparosc Endosc Percutan Tech 2014; 24(6):528–36.

79. Knight BC, Devitt PG, Watson DI, et al. Long-term efficacy of laparoscopic antireflux surgery on regression of Barrett's esophagus using BRAVO wireless pH monitoring: a prospective clinical cohort study. Ann Surg 2017;266(6):1000–5.

80. Leeds SG, Burdick JS, Fleshman JW. Endoluminal vacuum therapy for esophageal and upper intestinal anastomotic leaks. JAMA Surg 2016; 151(6):573.

81. Heits N, Stapel L, Reichert B, et al. Endoscopic endoluminal vacuum therapy in esophageal perforation. Ann Thorac Surg 2014;97(3):1029–35.

82. Bludau M, Hölscher AH, Herbold T, et al. Management of upper intestinal leaks using an endoscopic vacuum-assisted closure system (E-VAC). Surg Endosc 2014;28(3):896–901.

83. Wedemeyer J, Brangewitz M, Kubicka S, et al. Management of major postsurgical gastroesophageal intrathoracic leaks with an endoscopic vacuum-assisted closure system. Gastrointest Endosc 2010;71(2):382–6.

84. Ahrens M, Schulte T, Egberts J, et al. Drainage of esophageal leakage using endoscopic vacuum therapy: a prospective pilot study. Endoscopy 2010;42(9):693–8.

The Role of Novel Functional Probes in the Evaluation and Treatment of Esophageal Disease

Ezra N. Teitelbaum, MD, MEd[a],*, Christy M. Dunst, MD[b]

KEYWORDS

- Esophageal physiology • Gastroesophageal reflux disease • GERD • Achalasia
- Eosinophilic esophagitis • Functional lumen imaging probe • Mucosal impedance • Manometry

KEY POINTS

- Effective treatment of esophageal disease relies on a multifaceted evaluation of esophageal anatomy, physiology, and histology.
- The functional lumen imaging probe (FLIP) and mucosal impedance (MI) catheter are two novel technologies that can be used to evaluate esophageal function in a variety of disease states.
- FLIP uses impedance planimetry to measure the esophageal anatomy and determine the distensibility index (ie, resistance of the esophagus and esophagogastric junction to radial stretch).
- MI directly measures the impedance to electrical current through the esophageal mucosal surface. MI has been found to correlate with dilated intercellular spaces and other histologic changes caused by esophageal disease.

INTRODUCTION

The history of the treatment of esophageal disease over the last 100 years has been marked by technological advances that have greatly improved both diagnostic capabilities and the efficacy of therapeutic interventions. Advances in radiology, including contrast esophagram, CT, and PET, have allowed for a more granular assessment of esophageal anatomy and accurate detection and staging of malignant disease. In the late 1960s and 1970s, the development and rapid proliferation of flexible endoscopy radically altered the landscape of diagnosis and treatment of both benign and malignant esophageal disease.[1] Not only could the entire lumen of the esophagus and stomach be easily and safely visualized for assessment of anatomy and pathology but endoscopically based interventions could also be performed. Therapies, such as varied percutaneous endoscopic gastrostomy tube placement for feeding access, radiofrequency ablation for dysplastic Barrett esophagus and early cancer, band ligation of esophageal varices, and per-oral endoscopic myotomy (POEM) for achalasia, have dramatically reduced the invasiveness and morbidity of the treatment of these diseases.

The use of sensors and probes has also greatly enhanced our understanding of esophageal physiology and disease, and allowed for the accurate and objective diagnosis of a range of conditions. The introduction of conventional, and then high-resolution, manometry (HRM) allowed for the

Disclosures: The authors have nothing to disclose.
[a] Department of Surgery, Northwestern University Feinberg School of Medicine, 676 North St. Clair Street, Suite 650, Chicago, IL 60611, USA; [b] Foregut Surgeon, The Oregon Clinic, 4805 Northeast Glisan Street, Suite 6N60, Portland, OR 97213, USA
* Corresponding author.
E-mail address: Ezra.Teitelbaum@nm.org

scientific study of esophageal physiology and the nuanced diagnosis of a range of esophageal motility disorders, including achalasia.[2] The development of the 24-hour pH-monitoring catheter by Johnson and Demeester[3] in the 1970s enabled the objective assessment of gastroesophageal reflux (GER), allowing for a more precise and effective utilization of both medical and surgical therapies. The introduction of a wireless pH monitoring probe further reduced the patient discomfort associated with testing.[4]

In the past 10 years, the development and study of 2 novel esophageal measurement probes has further added to the armamentarium of clinicians evaluating and treating patients with esophageal disease. The functional lumen imaging probe (FLIP) and mucosal impedance (MI) catheter both use electrical impedance measurements to objectively assess properties of esophageal anatomy, physiology, and even histology. This review serves as an introduction to these two measurement devices and discusses the current evidence supporting their use in the diagnosis and treatment of a variety of esophageal diseases.

FUNCTIONAL LUMEN IMAGING PROBE
Functional Lumen Imaging Probe Technology

FLIP is a catheter-based device that is inserted transorally, usually with patients under moderate sedation or anesthesia in the setting of an upper endoscopy or surgical procedure. The distal end of the catheter shaft contains 16 electrode pairs spaced at fixed intervals (ranging 5–10 mm in current commercially available models [Crospon; Galway, Ireland]) over a span of 8 cm or 16 cm

(**Fig. 1**). The segment of the catheter that contains these electrodes is housed within an infinitely compliant plastic bag that can be variably inflated with saline solution using the device controls. Excitation electrodes at either end of the catheter emit a continuous low electric current, and impedance planimetry measurements are taken between each of the electrode pairs. These measurements are translated to cross-sectional areas (CSAs) at the level of each electrode pair using Ohm's law. These CSAs can then be combined to create a graphic representation of luminal anatomy that can be viewed in real time on the device display (**Fig. 2**).[5] A solid-state sensor measures pressure within the bag. FLIP has been most commonly used to measure the anatomy and function of the lower esophageal sphincter (LES) and esophageal body; but studies assessing its use for the upper esophageal sphincter, sphincter of Oddi, and anal sphincter have also been performed.[6–8] The most-studied FLIP measure of LES physiology is distensibility index (DI), which is calculated by dividing the minimum CSA (ie, narrowest point of the LES) by intrabag pressure. More recent studies have graphed CSA measurements (y-axis) over time (x-axis) to create FLIP topography plots, similar to the pressure topography plots used to display and analyze HRM measurements (**Fig. 3**). These topography graphs have enabled the use of FLIP to detect normal and abnormal esophageal contractions that occur in response to the volumetric distention caused by FLIP bag inflation, and represent a novel method for assessing esophageal motility.

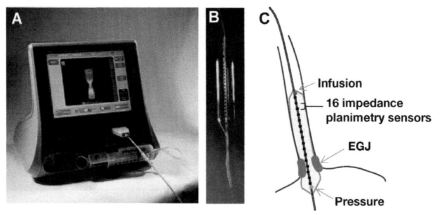

Fig. 1. The FLIP device and control console display (*A*) a graphic representation of esophageal lumen geometry. (*B*) A photograph and (*C*) cartoon of the FLIP measurement catheter are shown. The tip of the catheter contains 16 impedance planimetry electrodes and a pressor sensor, housed within a variably inflatable bag into which saline solution can be infused. EGJ, esophagogastric junction. (*From* Hirano I, Pandolfino JE, Boeckxstanes GE. Functional lumen imaging probe for management of esophageal disorders: expert review from the clinical practice updates committee of the AGA Institute. Clin Gastroenterol Hepatol 2017;15(3):325–34; with permission.)

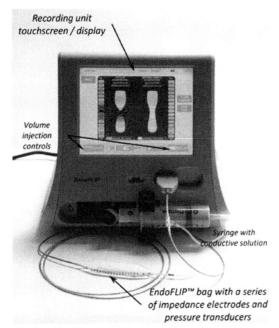

Recording unit touchscreen / display

Volume injection controls

Syringe with conductive solution

EndoFLIP™ bag with a series of impedance electrodes and pressure transducers

Fig. 2. The FLIP console displays a graphic representation of esophageal lumen geometry in real time as measurements are taken with the FLIP catheter. Touchscreen controls are used to variably inflate the FLIP catheter bag with saline solution. (*From* Kwiatek MA, Pandolfino JE, Hirano I, et al. Esophagogastric junction distensibility assessed with an endoscopic functional luminal imaging probe (EndoFLIP [Crospon; Galway, Ireland]). Gastrointest Endosc 2010;72(2):272–8; with permission.)

Achalasia

Achalasia is the most common primary esophageal motility disorder, resulting from an immune-mediated loss of esophageal inhibitory neurons. A resultant combined failure of LES relaxation and esophageal body peristalsis causes symptoms of dysphagia, regurgitation, chest pain, and weight loss.[9] Endoscopy is performed to rule out a mechanical source of obstruction, and the diagnosis is confirmed by HRM. Medical therapies are generally ineffective, and the mainstays of treatment are interventions designed to ablate the LES in order to allow for passive transit of food boluses into the stomach. Two such procedures, endoscopic pneumatic dilation and laparoscopic Heller myotomy, have been considered the standard of care for the past 20 years; a novel intervention POEM is rapidly gaining acceptance as a minimally invasive and durable alternative. Although HRM is considered the gold standard for the diagnosis of achalasia, less is known about the optimal evaluation of postintervention esophageal physiology. FLIP has recently been

introduced as an additional means of assessing patients with achalasia before, during, and after interventions.

Two landmark studies established the use of FLIP as a diagnostic tool for assessing LES physiology in patients with achalasia.[10,11] Both studies focused on the use of FLIP in assessing the efficacy of interventions for achalasia. Pandolfino and colleagues[10] performed FLIP measurements in 4 patient groups: healthy controls, patients with achalasia before treatment, and 2 groups of patients with achalasia after treatment (with either pneumatic dilation or surgical myotomy), those with a good symptom response and those with persistent symptoms. As expected, patients with untreated achalasia were found to have a much lower DI (ie, a less distensible or tighter) LES than healthy controls. However, a more interesting finding was that patients with a good response to treatment had a DI that was almost as high as healthy controls, whereas patients with a poor treatment response had a DI on par with the untreated achalasics. Furthermore, DI measurements using FLIP were better correlated with objective symptom scores in posttreatment patients than esophagogastric junction (EGJ) resting or relaxation pressures measured by HRM. In other words, FLIP measurements served as a better objective assessment of posttreatment physiology in patients with achalasia. A study by Rohof and colleagues[11] produced similar results, demonstrating that patients with untreated achalasia had a significantly lower DI than healthy controls (0.7 vs 6.3 mm^2/mm Hg; $P<.001$) and that posttreatment patients with symptomatic relief had higher DIs than those with poor clinical outcomes (4.4 vs 1.6 mm^2/mm Hg; $P = .001$). As with the study mentioned previously, FLIP DI was found to be more closely correlated with symptomatic outcomes than HRM pressures. The main driver of this result was a subset of patients who had reduced LES pressures after intervention but a poor clinical outcome. In these patients the DI was pathologically low, demonstrating the superiority of FLIP to HRM in the physiologic evaluation of patients with achalasia after pneumatic dilation or myotomy (**Fig. 4**). These studies established the use of FLIP in assessing outcomes after interventions for achalasia.

Based on this work, subsequent studies tested the utility of using FLIP as a measurement tool at the time of interventions for achalasia. The group at Northwestern University showed the feasibility of such assessments during both laparoscopic Heller myotomy and POEM procedures.[12] During this study, real-time FLIP measurements were performed during both procedures, showing a

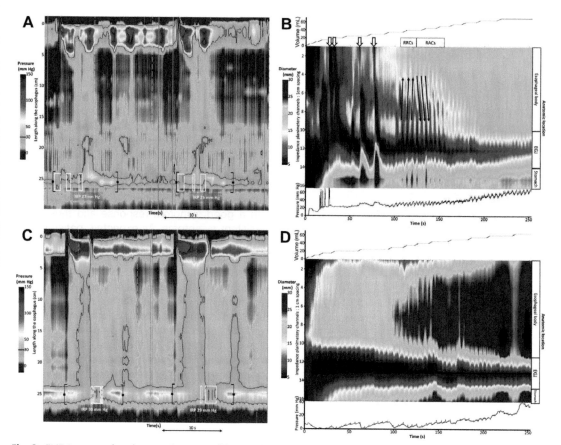

Fig. 3. FLIP topography plots can be created by graphing the length of the esophagus on the y-axis and time on the x-axis, with color representing luminal cross-sectional areas. These plots are similar to pressure topography plots (*A*) created using HRM. FLIP topography can be used to assess esophageal body motility (*B*) and can detect repetitive antegrade contractions (RACs) and repetitive retrograde contractions (RRCs) that are not seen on HRM (*C*). A FLIP topography plot (*D*) in a patient with type II achalasia shows an absence of RACs or RRCs. EGJ, esophagogastric junction. (*From* Carlson DA, Lin Z, Kahrilas PJ, et al. The functional lumen imaging probe detects esophageal contractility not observed with manometry in patients with achalasia. Gastroenterology 2015;149(7):1742–51; with permission.)

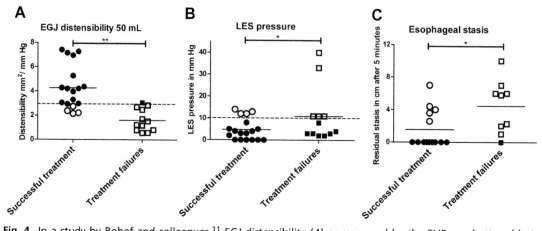

Fig. 4. In a study by Rohof and colleagues,[11] EGJ distensibility (*A*) as measured by the FLIP was better able to differentiate between patients with resolution and persistence of symptoms after procedural treatments for achalasia than either LES pressure on manometry (*B*) or esophageal stasis on esophagram (*C*) *Asterisks* denote *P*<.05. (*From* Rohof WO, Hirsch DP, Kessing BF, et al. Efficacy of treatment for patients with achalasia depends on the distensibility of the esophagogastric junction. Gastroenterology 2012;143(2):328–35; with permission.)

dramatic increase in DI as a result. Additionally, DI was assessed after each substep of these interventions (**Fig. 5**). During POEM, the steps of submucosal tunnel creation and myotomy were shown to both result in independent increases in DI. During laparoscopic Heller, performing the myotomy greatly increased DI (from a mean of 1.3 to 5.2 mm^2/mm Hg; $P<.001$), whereas subsequent creation of a partial fundoplication lowered DI (from 5.2 to 3.9 mm^2/mm Hg; $P<.01$). These results provided the first support for the use of FLIP as an intraoperative calibration tool. Theoretically, DI measurements could be used to ensure that adequacy of the myotomy in increasing LES compliance. During Heller myotomy with partial fundoplication, FLIP could then be used to tailor the fundoplication to verify that an adequate antireflux barrier had been created without excessively tightening the EGJ, which could result in postoperative dysphagia.

This concept was expanded on in 2 later studies in which sequential FLIP measurements were performed as the myotomy was created in increments during Heller and POEM.[13,14] In the first study, a short myotomy across the LES was created from 2 cm proximal to the EGJ to 3 cm distal to the EGJ and onto the stomach. After an initial FLIP measurement was taken, the myotomy was extended proximally to a total of 6 cm proximal to the EGJ. Interestingly, this proximal extension was necessary to normalize DI during laparoscopic Heller myotomy, but the shorter myotomy confined to the LES was sufficient in POEM

procedures.[13] A later study explored a similar question, this time extending the myotomy in an incremental fashion from proximal to distal during POEM procedures. These results showed that a myotomy across the LES and a further extension to 2 cm distal to the EGJ both increased DI significantly, whereas a subsequent extension to 3 cm distal to the EGJ did not further increase in DI.[14] During both of these studies there was a sizable degree of variability in DI measurements between individual patients at each of the operative time points. This finding suggests that rather than identifying an ideal myotomy length that applies to all patients, a better use of FLIP would be as a real-time calibration tool to tailor the proximal and distal myotomy length to each patient's unique physiologic requirements.

Based on the findings that DI correlates well with postintervention symptoms and FLIP can be used to measure DI in real time during laparoscopic Heller myotomy and POEM, subsequent research sought to establish whether intraoperative FLIP measurements can predict eventual clinical outcomes. During achalasia interventions, relief of symptoms, such as dysphagia and regurgitation, depends on successful ablation of the LES. However, if the compliance of the LES is increased too much, it could theoretically result in a higher incidence of postintervention iatrogenic GER. One study compared intraoperative FLIP measurements taken at the conclusion of both Heller myotomy and POEM procedures with outcomes in regard to both achalasia and GER symptoms.[15]

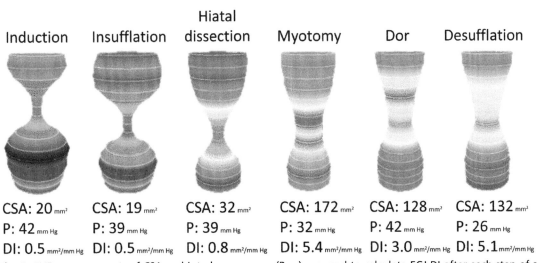

Induction	Insufflation	Hiatal dissection	Myotomy	Dor	Desufflation
CSA: 20 mm²	CSA: 19 mm²	CSA: 32 mm²	CSA: 172 mm²	CSA: 128 mm²	CSA: 132 mm²
P: 42 mm Hg	P: 39 mm Hg	P: 39 mm Hg	P: 32 mm Hg	P: 42 mm Hg	P: 26 mm Hg
DI: 0.5 mm²/mm Hg	DI: 0.5 mm²/mm Hg	DI: 0.8 mm²/mm Hg	DI: 5.4 mm²/mm Hg	DI: 3.0 mm²/mm Hg	DI: 5.1 mm²/mm Hg

Fig. 5. FLIP measurements of CSA and intrabag pressure (Pres) are used to calculate EGJ DI after each step of a laparoscopic Heller myotomy with Dor fundoplication. A large increase in DI is seen after myotomy, and then a smaller decrease in DI occurs after creation of the Dor fundoplication. (*From* Teitelbaum EN, Boris L, Arafat FO, et al. Comparison of esophagogastric junction distensibility changes during POEM and Heller myotomy using intraoperative FLIP. Surg Endosc 2013;27(12):4547–55; with permission.)

During Heller myotomy, the only 2 patients with ending DI less than 3 both had poor symptomatic outcomes; across all Heller patients, the final intraoperative DI correlated with postoperative achalasia symptoms, as measured by the Eckardt symptom score.[16] Additionally, patients with a higher final DI were more likely to go on to have symptoms suggestive of iatrogentic GER. Compiling these two results, the investigators were able to determine a sweet spot range of the final DI: 4.5 to 8.5 mm^2/mm Hg. Patients who ended their procedure within this ideal range had optimal outcomes (minimal achalasia and GER symptoms) in 88% of cases, as opposed to only 47% of patients whose final DI was either greater than or less than this range.

Another study by Ngamruengphong and colleagues[17] added evidence to the predictive validity of FLIP measurements taken during POEM for the treatment of achalasia. The investigators found that patients with superior relief of achalasia symptoms (defined as an Eckardt score <3) had a higher mean LES CSA as compared with those with poor clinical outcomes. Additionally, patients with reflux esophagitis on follow-up endoscopy had higher CSA. These data support the concept that during operations for achalasia, a certain distensibility threshold must be met in order to ensure adequate relief of dysphagia. Conversely, too high a final DI may predispose patients to postoperative GER and esophagitis. Using FLIP during such operations could potentially serve as a quality-control measure to evaluate DI as the procedure progresses and tailor the myotomy and fundoplication to ensure that each operation ends with a DI in the ideal range.

A related study has shown a similar relationship between postintervention DI and symptomatic outcomes in patients undergoing pneumatic dilation for the treatment of achalasia.[18] Wu and colleagues[18] performed FLIP measurements before and after dilation in 54 patients. In patients with an immediate symptomatic response to dilation, DI increased by a mean of 4.5 mm^2/mm Hg, whereas in patients without symptomatic improvement, there was no significant change in DI. When evaluated as a continuous variable, DI was highly predictive of the clinical response to dilation, with an area under the curve of 0.89. A DI increase threshold of 1.8 mm^2/mm Hg was predictive of a good clinical outcome with 87% accuracy. Although pneumatic dilation to a fixed diameter (ie, 30, 35, or 40 mm) does not allow for calibration using intraprocedure FLIP, postdilation DI could be used to prognosticate and predict the need for repeat dilations at larger diameters or consideration for transition to alternative interventions, such as laparoscopic Heller or POEM, in patients who do not achieve an adequate distensibility increase.

Although initial investigations into the use of FLIP in patients with achalasia focused on its utility in the assessment of postintervention symptoms and measurement during these procedures, more recent studies have expanded the role of FLIP to the point of diagnosis. HRM measures LES pressures in response to swallowing and esophageal body contractility, and abnormalities in both are required to establish a diagnosis of achalasia. The studies using FLIP described previously only examined its ability to evaluate the LES. More recent work has expanded FLIP measurements to assess esophageal body activity in response to distention, by using a FLIP catheter with a longer 16 cm impedance electrode array and bag, compared with the 8 cm catheters used in prior studies. In addition to measuring LES DI at set time points, FLIP measurements have been recorded longitudinally over time to create FLIP topography plots similar to the pressure topography plots (ie, Clause plots) used to display and analyze HRM measurements (**Fig. 6**).

Carlson and colleagues[19] used such a graphical analysis and observed that FLIP can detect motility of the esophageal body (both normal and pathologic) in addition to LES distensibility. In healthy controls, inflation of the FLIP bag results in forward propagating peristaltic waves, similar to those seen with swallowing on HRM (**Fig. 7**). These waves occur in clusters, and the investigators termed them repetitive, antegrade contractions (RACs). Conversely, in patients with achalasia (particularly type III) and other esophageal motility disorders, FLIP distension produces repetitive, retrograde contractions (RRCs), a finding without a correlate on HRM. By combining the findings of LES DI and esophageal body contractility (absent, RACs, or RRCs), FLIP can now be used to fully assess esophageal physiology in a way that may compliment HRM. When HRM and FLIP were compared in 145 patients with dysphagia, 95% of patients with an abnormal HRM also had a corresponding abnormal FLIP, including all patients with an HRM diagnosis of achalasia. However, in the patients with a normal HRM, 50% had an abnormality seen on FLIP topography. These findings were used to create an algorithm for the analysis of FLIP measurements (**Fig. 8**), similar to the way in which the Chicago Classification is used to categorize patients based on HRM.[2] If validated in future studies, this classification system using FLIP could go on to serve as a complement, or even an eventual replacement, to the use of HRM for the evaluation

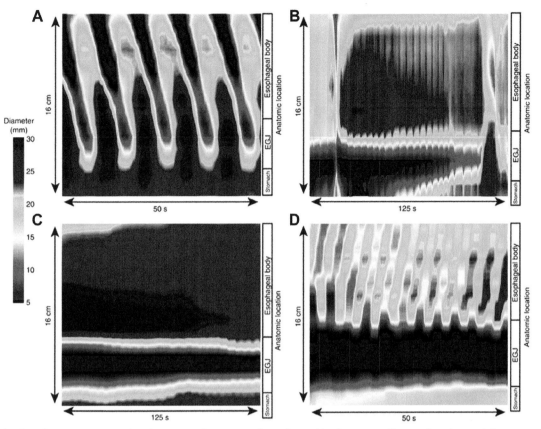

Fig. 6. Using FLIP topography plots, several patterns of esophageal body contractility can be observed. In asymptomatic controls, distention with the FLIP bag produces (A) repetitive, antegrade contractions (RACs). Patients with EGJ outflow obstruction with ineffective esophageal motility showed (B) esophageal contractility without RACs or repetitive, retrograde contractions (RRCs). Patients with type I achalasia typically have (C) elevated EGJ distensibility without any form of esophageal body contraction. Patients with type III achalasia often demonstrate (D) RRCs. (*Reprinted by* permission from Springer Nature. *From* Carlson DA, Kahrilas PJ, Lin Z, et al. Evaluation of esophageal motility utilizing the functional lumen imaging probe. The American Journal of Gastroenterology 2016;111:1726–35.)

and diagnosis of patients with nonobstructive dysphagia.

Eosinophilic Esophagitis

Eosinophilic esophagitis (EoE) is a food-allergen-driven immune-mediated disease of the esophagus that results in chronic eosinophil predominate inflammation.[20] Over time, this leads to fibrosis and stricturing of the esophageal body, causing symptoms of dysphagia and food impaction. Visual findings on endoscopy can be present, and the diagnosis is confirmed by identification of eosinophils on histology from esophageal biopsies. Treatment consists of a trial of gastric acid suppression with a proton-pump inhibitor (PPI) and, if unsuccessful, progression to topical steroids (ingested orally) and/or structured food elimination diets. Endoscopic dilation is used

when fibrotic strictures occur as a result of long-standing inflammation. FLIP has recently been used to measure luminal distensibility and esophageal motility in patients with EoE and may serve as a useful adjunct measure in the diagnosis, prognostication, and assessment of treatment efficacy in such patients.

An initial study by Kwiatek and colleagues[21] evaluated FLIP measurements performed in 33 patients with EoE and 15 healthy controls. Not surprisingly, the patients with EoE were found to have a lower DI than the healthy controls; but interestingly, the histologic eosinophil count in the patients with EoE did not correlate with FLIP DI. A subsequent study of patients with EoE demonstrated that the severity of esophageal rings (ie, EoE strictures) was associated with lower distensibility as measured by FLIP (**Fig. 9**).[22] These findings suggest that FLIP is a measure of chronic

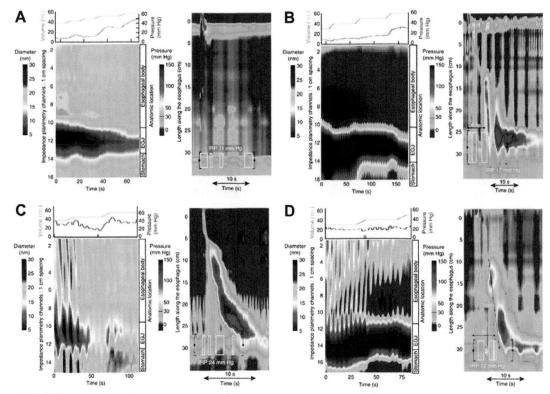

Fig. 7. FLIP topography plots were compared with HRM pressure topography plots in several patients. In a patient with type I achalasia FLIP topography (*A*) showed abnormal distensibility and absent contractility, whereas HRM had borderline relaxation pressure. In a patient (*B*) with esophagogastric outflow obstruction (EGJOO) but partially preserved peristalsis on HRM, FLIP showed elevated distensibility and no normal esophageal body contractility, suggesting a diagnosis of achalasia. Conversely, another patient (*C*) with EGJOO on HRM showed normal distensibility and repetitive, antegrade contractions on FLIP, making achalasia unlikely. Finally, a patient (*D*) with dysphagia had a normal HRM but elevated distensibility and repetitive, retrograde contractions on FLIP, suggesting that FLIP may be the more sensitive diagnostic test for esophageal motility disorders in certain patients. (*Reprinted by* permission from Springer Nature. *From* Carlson DA, Kahrilas PJ, Lin Z, et al. Evaluation of esophageal motility utilizing the functional lumen imaging probe. The American Journal of Gastroenterology 2016;111:1726–35.)

fibrosis and stricturing rather than acute inflammation in patients with EoE. Following from this, another study showed that FLIP measurements were able to predict the occurrence of food impaction and the need for endoscopic dilation during follow-up in patients with EoE.[23] In addition to prognostication, FLIP may be useful in evaluating the treatment effect in patients with EoE. A study by Carlson and colleagues[24] demonstrated that esophageal distensibility increased after initiation of EoE treatment (with topical steroids, food elimination diet, or PPI) without esophageal dilation. This finding suggests that although FLIP distensibility is primarily a measure of fibrosis and stricturing in patients with EoE, this fibrosis can potentially be remodeled as a result of medical or dietary therapy. If FLIP measurements are shown to be an effective objective marker of the efficacy of such treatments, it could replace the use of histologic analysis of multiple interval biopsies, which are costly and time consuming to obtain and evaluate.

Gastroesophageal Reflux Disease

GER disease (GERD) is an extremely common condition resulting from the failure of the mechanical barrier of the LES to prevent retrograde reflux of acidic gastric secretions into the esophagus.[25] It causes symptoms of heartburn and regurgitation and over time can lead to the formation of peptic strictures and the metaplastic conversion of esophageal squamous to intestinal columnar mucosa (ie, Barrett esophagus), which is a risk factor for the development of esophageal adenocarcinoma. Empiric treatment is often initiated based on symptoms alone, but 24-hour pH monitoring is the gold standard for establishing an objective diagnosis.

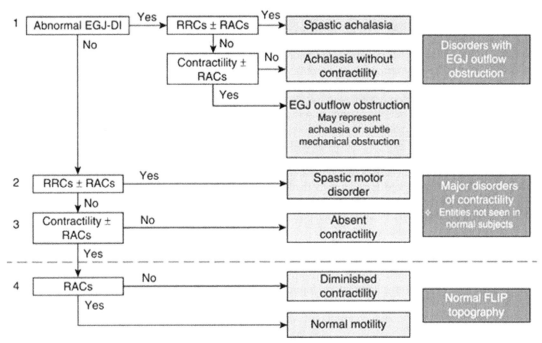

Fig. 8. A proposed algorithm for using FLIP topography to diagnose esophageal motility orders. EGJ-DI, EGJ distensibility. (*Reprinted by* permission from Springer Nature. *From* Carlson DA, Kahrilas PJ, Lin Z, et al. Evaluation of esophageal motility utilizing the functional lumen imaging probe. The American Journal of Gastroenterology 2016;111:1726–35.)

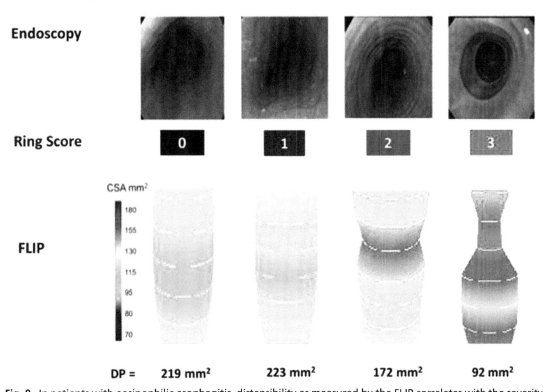

Fig. 9. In patients with eosinophilic esophagitis, distensibility as measured by the FLIP correlates with the severity of esophageal stenosis seen on upper endoscopy. *DP,* distensibility plateau. (*From* Chen JW, Pandolfino JE, Lin Z, et al. Severity of endoscopically identified esophageal rings correlates with reduced esophageal distensibility in eosinophilic esophagitis. Endoscopy 2016;48(9):794–801; with permission.)

Medical therapy with PPIs forms the mainstay of palliative treatment of GERD; surgical therapy, traditionally a laparoscopic fundoplication, is offered to patients who desire freedom from long-term medication dependence, have symptoms that are refractory to PPI therapy, or have complications of GERD, such as stricture, that develop or progress despite medical management. As LES functional integrity in the face of postprandial gastric distension is key to the prevention of GER, it follows that LES distensibility as measured by FLIP may be a valid metric in the evaluation of patients with GERD. Such research is still in its infancy; but there is reason to think that FLIP may serve as a valuable adjunct physiologic measure in the diagnosis, treatment, and post-intervention evaluation of patients with GERD.

In an early study by Kwiatek and colleagues,[5] FLIP measurements at the EGJ were performed in healthy controls and patients with symptoms consistent with GERD. The investigators found that the patients with GERD had a LES DI that was twice that of healthy controls (8 vs 4 mm^2/mm Hg; $P<.05$). The was no correlation between FLIP distensibility measurements and endoscopically visualized Hill grade[26] of the EGJ flap valve. This finding suggests that although FLIP has the capacity to measure the compliance of the LES, it does not detect all the anatomic aspects of the EGJ that contribute to the prevention of GER. Another study showed that after undergoing fundoplication for treatment of GERD, patients had lower DI than healthy controls.[27] This finding formed the basis for potential intraoperative use of FLIP in order to calibrate the fundoplication.

DeHaan and colleagues[28] performed such a study in which intraoperative FLIP measurements were taken in 2 sets of patients: those undergoing compete, 360° fundoplication (ie, Nissen fundoplication) and others during partial posterior fundoplication (ie, Toupet fundoplication). They found that Toupet fundoplication resulted in a higher (ie, less constricted) final DI. In prior studies, Toupet fundoplication has been shown to result in fewer postoperative symptoms of dysphagia and gas bloating when compared with Nissen.[29] The difference in FLIP distensibility between the two fundoplications raises the possibility that such intraoperative measurements could be used to calibrate wrap tightness in order to avoid postoperative dysphagia. However, further work is needed to correlate intraoperative FLIP measurements with postoperative symptomatic and physiologic outcomes in patients undergoing antireflux surgery before the technology can be applied during surgery on a routine basis.

MUCOSAL IMPENDENCE
Mucosal Impendence Technology

As opposed to FLIP, which uses impedance planimetry measurements to calculate interval CSAs in order to evaluate esophageal luminal anatomy, MI uses electrical tissue impedance spectroscopy technology to measure the surface bioelectrical properties of the esophageal mucosa itself. These measurements can evaluate histologic and functional aspects of the mucosa and its response to disease states. The MI probe is a narrow, flexible catheter that fits through the working channel of a standard gastroscope (**Fig. 10**).[30] Its tip contains impedance electrodes; when the probe is advanced to contact the esophagus, these electrodes measure the resistance to the flow of an electrical current passing between the electrodes across the mucosal surface.[31] MI can be altered by changes in mucosal histology, such as the presence of dilated intercellular spaces (DIS). Such DIS can form as a response to acid exposure in patients with GERD[32]; thus, MI may serve as an effective and efficient measure of the histologic response of the esophageal mucosa to GER and other disease states. The ability to perform MI measurements in real time during diagnostic and therapeutic upper endoscopy makes the technology an attractive alternative to costly, time-consuming, and/or uncomfortable diagnostic

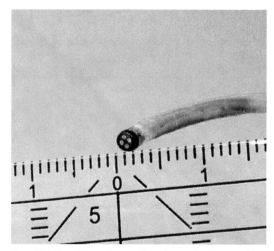

Fig. 10. The MI catheter fits through the working channel of a flexible gastroscope. Its tip, shown in this image, contains electrodes that measure tissue impedance when placed into contact with the esophageal mucosa. (*From* Weijenborg PW, Rohof WOA, Akkermans LMA, et al. Electrical tissue impedance spectroscopy: a novel device to measure esophageal mucosal integrity changes during endoscopy. Neurogastroenterol Motil 2013;25(7):57–8; with permission.)

tests, such as tissue biopsy histology and 24-hour pH monitoring.

Clinical Uses of Mucosal Impendence

Several early studies have laid the theoretic groundwork for the use of MI in the diagnosis and management of GERD and EoE. Saritas Yuksel and colleagues[33] performed MI measurements in patients with GERD confirmed by 24-hour pH monitoring and in healthy controls. They found that MI values at 2 cm proximal to the EGJ were lower in patients with GERD (2096 Ω vs 3607 Ω; $P<.01$). Additionally, in patients with GERD there was a gradient of MI that increased as the probe was moved from distal to proximal in the esophageal body. In the area of erosive esophagitis, the MI values were significantly lower than in noninflamed mucosa. Taken together, these results suggest that MI can detect mucosal changes resulting from GER and additionally grade the severity of those changes. In a subsequent study, MI measurements were compared with 24-hour pH monitoring results in their ability to predict the presence of erosive esophagitis on endoscopy. MI was found to have superior specificity and positive predictive values (95% and 96%, respectively) as compared with pH monitoring (64% and 40%), whereas the sensitivity and negative predictive values of the tests were similar.[34] If these results can be validated in future studies, MI could potentially supplant 24-hour pH monitoring as the test of choice for objective confirmation of the presence of pathologic GER because of its ease of application during diagnostic upper endoscopy.

Similar work has evaluated the utility of MI measurements in patients with EoE. Katzka and colleagues[35] performed endoscopic MI measurements and esophageal biopsies on 3 groups: healthy controls, patients with active EoE, and patients with inactive EoE. They found that MI was significantly lower in patients with active EoE (defined by >15 eosinophils per high-power field on biopsy) when compared with healthy controls and patients with inactive, or posttreatment, EoE. There was excellent overall correlation between MI and the number of eosinophils on biopsy; MI was able to distinguish between active and inactive disease with a sensitivity and specificity of 90% and 91%, respectively, using an impedance cutoff of 2300 Ω. Furthermore, MI correlated well with the degree of DIS seen on histology. These data suggest that although FLIP may be a surrogate marker of chronic fibrosis and stricture in patients with EoE, MI is able to detect active

eosinophil-mediated inflammation. This finding supports the ongoing study, and potential future clinical use, of both FLIP and MI as complementary objective assessments in such patients to monitor disease progression and treatment response.

SUMMARY

A multifaceted evaluation of anatomy, physiology, and histology is essential to the medical and surgical treatment of esophageal disease. Technological advancements have allowed for a more nuanced assessment of each of these components of esophageal function, and this in turn has allowed for more targeted and effective therapies that are tailored to individual patients' specific conditions. The recent introduction of FLIP and MI into the armamentarium of the esophagologist has broadened the options for such evaluation and application of personalized medicine to the esophagus. Although further study is needed to validate the early results described in this review and more clearly define the role of these technologies in patient assessment, it is clear that FLIP and MI each offer a novel and exciting method to better understand esophageal function in normal and disease states.

REFERENCES

1. Sivak MV. Gastrointestinal endoscopy: past and future. Gut 2006;55:1061–4.
2. Kahrilas PJ, Bredenoord AJ, Fox M, et al. The Chicago Classification of esophageal motility disorders, v3.0. Neurogastroenterol Motil 2015;27:160–74.
3. Johnson LF, Demeester TR. Twenty-four-hour pH monitoring of the distal esophagus. A quantitative measure of gastroesophageal reflux. Am J Gastroenterol 1974;62:325–32.
4. Richter JE, Pandolfino JE, Vela MF, et al. Utilization of wireless pH monitoring technologies: a summary of the proceedings from the esophageal diagnostic working group. Dis Esophagus 2013;26:755–65.
5. Kwiatek MA, Pandolfino JE, Hirano I, et al. Esophagogastric junction distensibility assessed with an endoscopic functional luminal imaging probe (EndoFLIP). Gastrointest Endosc 2010;72:272–8.
6. Sorensen G, Liao D, Lundby L, et al. Distensibility of the anal canal in patients with idiopathic fecal incontinence: a study with the Functional Lumen Imaging Probe. Neurogastroenterol Motil 2014;26: 255–63.
7. Regan J, Walshe M, Rommel N, et al. A new evaluation of the upper esophageal sphincter using the functional lumen imaging probe: a preliminary report. Dis Esophagus 2013;26:117–23.

8. Kunwald P, Drewes AM, Kjaer D, et al. A new distensibility technique to measure sphincter of Oddi function. Neurogastroenterol Motil 2010;22: 978–83. e253.

9. Boeckxstaens GE, Zaninotto G, Richter JE. Achalasia. Lancet 2014;383:83–93.

10. Pandolfino JE, de Ruigh A, Nicodeme F, et al. Distensibility of the esophagogastric junction assessed with the functional lumen imaging probe (FLIP) in achalasia patients. Neurogastroenterol Motil 2013;25:496–501.

11. Rohof WO, Hirsch DP, Kessing BF, et al. Efficacy of treatment for patients with achalasia depends on the distensibility of the esophagogastric junction. Gastroenterology 2012;143:328–35.

12. Teitelbaum EN, Boris L, Arafat FO, et al. Comparison of esophagogastric junction distensibility changes during POEM and Heller myotomy using intraoperative FLIP. Surg Endosc 2013;27:4547–55.

13. Teitelbaum EN, Soper NJ, Pandolfino JE, et al. An extended proximal esophageal myotomy is necessary to normalize EGJ distensibility during Heller myotomy for achalasia, but not POEM. Surg Endosc 2014;28:2840–7.

14. Teitelbaum EN, Sternbach JM, El Khoury R, et al. The effect of incremental distal gastric myotomy lengths on EGJ distensibility during POEM for achalasia. Surg Endosc 2016;30:745–50.

15. Teitelbaum EN, Soper NJ, Pandolfino JE, et al. Esophagogastric junction distensibility measurements during Heller myotomy and POEM for achalasia predict postoperative symptomatic outcomes. Surg Endosc 2015;29:522–8.

16. Eckardt VF. Clinical presentations and complications of achalasia. Gastrointest Endosc Clin N Am 2001; 11:281–92, vi.

17. Ngamruengphong S, von Rahden BH, Filser J, et al. Intraoperative measurement of esophagogastric junction cross-sectional area by impedance planimetry correlates with clinical outcomes of peroral endoscopic myotomy for achalasia: a multicenter study. Surg Endosc 2016;30:2886–94.

18. Wu PI, Szczesniak MM, Craig PI, et al. Novel intraprocedural distensibility measurement accurately predicts immediate outcome of pneumatic dilatation for idiopathic achalasia. Am J Gastroenterol 2018; 113(2):205–12.

19. Carlson DA, Kahrilas PJ, Lin Z, et al. Evaluation of esophageal motility utilizing the functional lumen imaging probe. Am J Gastroenterol 2016;111: 1726–35.

20. Chen JW, Kao JY. Eosinophilic esophagitis: update on management and controversies. BMJ 2017;359: j4482.

21. Kwiatek MA, Hirano I, Kahrilas PJ, et al. Mechanical properties of the esophagus in eosinophilic esophagitis. Gastroenterology 2011;140:82–90.

22. Chen JW, Pandolfino JE, Lin Z, et al. Severity of endoscopically identified esophageal rings correlates with reduced esophageal distensibility in eosinophilic esophagitis. Endoscopy 2016;48:794–801.

23. Nicodeme F, Hirano I, Chen J, et al. Esophageal distensibility as a measure of disease severity in patients with eosinophilic esophagitis. Clin Gastroenterol Hepatol 2013;11:1101–7.e1.

24. Carlson DA, Hirano I, Zalewski A, et al. Improvement in esophageal distensibility in response to medical and diet therapy in eosinophilic esophagitis. Clin Transl Gastroenterol 2017;8:e119.

25. Kahrilas PJ. Clinical practice. Gastroesophageal reflux disease. N Engl J Med 2008;359:1700–7.

26. Hill LD, Kozarek RA, Kraemer SJ, et al. The gastroesophageal flap valve: in vitro and in vivo observations. Gastrointest Endosc 1996;44:541–7.

27. Kwiatek MA, Kahrilas K, Soper NJ, et al. Esophagogastric junction distensibility after fundoplication assessed with a novel functional luminal imaging probe. J Gastrointest Surg 2010;14:268–76.

28. DeHaan RK, Davila D, Frelich MJ, et al. Esophagogastric junction distensibility is greater following Toupet compared to Nissen fundoplication. Surg Endosc 2017;31:193–8.

29. Broeders JA, Mauritz FA, Ahmed Ali U, et al. Systematic review and meta-analysis of laparoscopic Nissen (posterior total) versus Toupet (posterior partial) fundoplication for gastro-oesophageal reflux disease. Br J Surg 2010;97:1318–30.

30. Weijenborg PW, Rohof WO, Akkermans LM, et al. Electrical tissue impedance spectroscopy: a novel device to measure esophageal mucosal integrity changes during endoscopy. Neurogastroenterol Motil 2013;25:574–8. e457–8.

31. Jones DM, Smallwood RH, Hose DR, et al. Modelling of epithelial tissue impedance measured using three different designs of probe. Physiol Meas 2003;24: 605–23.

32. Caviglia R, Ribolsi M, Maggiano N, et al. Dilated intercellular spaces of esophageal epithelium in nonerosive reflux disease patients with physiological esophageal acid exposure. Am J Gastroenterol 2005;100:543–8.

33. Saritas Yuksel E, Higginbotham T, Slaughter JC, et al. Use of direct, endoscopic-guided measurements of mucosal impedance in diagnosis of gastroesophageal reflux disease. Clin Gastroenterol Hepatol 2012;10:1110–6.

34. Ates F, Yuksel ES, Higginbotham T, et al. Mucosal impedance discriminates GERD from non-GERD conditions. Gastroenterology 2015;148:334–43.

35. Katzka DA, Ravi K, Geno DM, et al. Endoscopic mucosal impedance measurements correlate with eosinophilia and dilation of intercellular spaces in patients with eosinophilic esophagitis. Clin Gastroenterol Hepatol 2015;13:1242–8.e1.

The Role of Intraoperative Fluorescence Imaging During Esophagectomy

Simon R. Turner, MD, MEd, FRCSC[a],
Daniela R. Molena, MD[b],*

KEYWORDS

• Esophagectomy • Esophageal cancer • Fluorescence imaging • Indocyanine green • Perfusion
• Anastomotic leak • Sentinel node • Chylothorax

KEY POINTS

• Fluorescence imaging, commonly with indocyanine green (ICG) has the potential to address several challenges encountered in esophagectomy.
• Intravascular injection of ICG allows visualization of conduit vascular supply and assessment of perfusion to potentially reduce anastomotic leaks.
• Peritumoral injection of ICG may allow identification of sentinel nodes in esophagectomy, although the oncologic value of this technique is unknown.
• Intralymphatic injection of ICG allows the visualization of the thoracic duct, which may allow preservation of the duct and easier ligation for duct injuries.

BACKGROUND

In recent years, advances in both technique and technology have aimed to minimize the morbidity associated with esophagectomy and improve oncologic outcomes. Most notably, the introduction of minimally invasive esophagectomy and the application of robotic surgical technology have offered the chance to improve perioperative and long-term results. However, despite these innovations, several stubborn challenges remain unresolved in esophageal resection, including the assessment of conduit perfusion in preventing anastomotic leaks, adequate lymphadenectomy, and prevention of thoracic duct injuries. Intraoperative fluorescence imaging (FI) is an emerging technology that may have the potential to address each of these challenges.

FI involves the injection of a small quantity of fluorescent dye into the patient at a specified time in the operation. Most often, a specialized camera is used with a separate FI light source and sensor. The FI light source emits light at a wavelength tuned to excite the fluorescent dye, which in turn releases a known wavelength of light back to the FI sensor.[1] The image generated by the fluorescence can be viewed on its own or superimposed on a standard laparoscopic/thoracoscopic image, thus highlighting, in real-time, organ perfusion and areas of relevant anatomy, such as blood supply and lymphatic drainage. The dye most often used in esophageal surgery is indocyanine green (ICG). In the past, fluorescein was used in surgical applications because of the ability to see the emitted fluorescence with the naked eye,

Disclosures: Dr S.R. Turner has nothing to disclose. Dr D.R. Molena reports speaking engagements with Novadaq technologies.
[a] Division of Thoracic Surgery, University of Alberta, 416 CSC, 10240 Kingsway Avenue, Edmonton, Alberta, T5H 3V9, Canada; [b] Thoracic Surgery Service, Memorial Sloan Kettering Cancer Center, 1275 York Avenue, New York, NY 10065, USA
* Corresponding author.
E-mail address: molenad@mskcc.org

without the use of a specialized camera. However, ICG has the advantage of better visualization of deeper tissues than fluorescein[1] and has gained recent popularity. ICG is safe, approved for use in humans, and has extensive history of use in ophthalmology, cardiac and vascular surgery, plastic and reconstructive surgery, oncologic surgery, and cardiology.[1] Adverse reactions may be possible in patients with allergies to iodine or shellfish.[2] Several FI camera options for ICG exist on the market, including the SPY and Pinpoint systems from Novadaq (Novadaq, Ontario, Canada) and the HyperEye Medical System (Mizuho Ikakogyo Co, Tokyo, Japan), both of which combine a standard laparoscope/thoracoscope with an ICG camera, and the Da Vinci robotic surgical system (Intuitive Surgical, Sunnyvale, CA), which has built-in ICG imaging capabilities.

ASSESSMENT OF GASTRIC CONDUIT PERFUSION IN PREVENTING ANASTOMOTIC LEAKS

Chief among the challenges faced by esophageal surgeons is the risk of anastomotic leak, the most significant of the common complications after this operation. Leak rates remain a disappointingly high 10% or more and are associated with increased perioperative mortality, morbidity, and length of stay.[3] The high rate of leaks relative to other types of anastomoses is related, at least in part, to the need to rely on a single arterial supply for the transposed stomach that originates distally, such that the area used for the anastomosis is by definition the most ischemic part of the conduit, perfused entirely by submucosal vascular channels.

Classically, assessment of the gastric conduit's perfusion has depended on fairly unreliable measures such as visual inspection of the stomach's color and the palpation of temperature and pulse. Even the use of Doppler ultrasound technology only provides information about the macrocirculation, while it is the microcirculation that is truly critical to anastomotic healing. Intraoperative FI, on the other hand, provides qualitative and quantitative information about both micro- and macrocirculatory health of the gastric conduit. FI dye can be administered intravenously either during conduit preparation in the abdominal phase of the operation and/or before performing the anastomosis in the chest or neck. By observing the speed with which the conduit enhances as well as any areas of demarcation in the conduit, the overall perfusion can be assessed and an optimal location for performing the anastomosis can be selected. This is commonly done qualitatively,

with a gross visual assessment of the fluorescence of the conduit, although quantitative measures can be performed. The speed of fluorescence flow can be measured and has been associated with anastomotic leak rates.[4] External software (Luminview, Mizuho Ikakogyo Co., Tokyo, Japan) is also available, which allows quantitative measurement of fluorescence intensity,[5] and newer versions of FI camera systems now feature quantitative assessments built in (Novadaq, Ontario, Canada).

One of the largest series reporting the use of FI in assessing conduit perfusion is by Zehetner and colleagues.[2] In this study, 150 consecutive esophagectomies with cervical esophagogastric anastomosis were performed with ICG assessment of the conduit intraoperatively in the abdominal phase. An assessment was made as to whether the conduit had rapid and robust perfusion or evidence of a demarcation, with an area of poor perfusion. In cases with poor perfusion a stitch was placed at the site of demarcation and an attempt was made to place the anastomosis proximal to the stitch (closer to the origin of the right gastroepiploic artery), although this was not always possible. Eighty-four (66%) patients had an area of demarcation with poor perfusion distally in the fundus noted. Twenty-nine of these patients had the anastomosis performed proximal to the demarcation (closer to the artery), 49 were performed distally (toward the fundus), and 6 had delayed reconstruction at a second phase. Patients with anastomosis placed distally had a higher risk of leak compared with anastomoses proximal to the demarcation and those with no demarcation noted (45% vs 2%, $P<.0001$). In multivariate analysis, anastomosis in an area of poor graft perfusion was the only significant predictor of a leak. Similarly, Campbell, and colleagues[6] noted a decrease in their anastomotic leak rate from 20% to 0% ($P = .007$) after the introduction of both Doppler ultrasound and ICG FI to assess their gastric conduits.

ICG has also been used to help identify the route of the right gastroepiploic artery in order to better protect it during division of the greater omentum,[7] as well as to visualize the intramural blood supply of gastric, colonic, and jejunal conduits[8] or the vascularity of omental flaps used for anastomotic reinforcement.[9] The authors' colleagues at Memorial Sloan Kettering Cancer Center noted that the use of ICG FI during robotic esophagectomy allowed improved visualization of the right gastroepiploic artery and the identification of "otherwise unvisualized small transverse vessels between the termination of the vascular arcade and the...short gastric arteries."[10] Kitagawa and colleagues[11] demonstrated a nonstatistically significant decreased leak rate from 17.9% to 4.4% ($P = .2$) with the use of FI to denote intramural arterial arcade anatomy before the creation of the gastric conduit. Lastly, Kamyia and colleagues[12] used videos of ICG FI to retrospectively evaluate the perfusion of 26 free jejunal grafts and found that quantitative measures of poor perfusion were associated with the 5 patients in the series who had a venous anastomotic failure.

SENTINEL NODE MAPPING

Another recalcitrant challenge in esophageal surgery relates to oncologic outcomes. Long-term survival rates with esophageal cancer are low even after trimodality therapy.[13] This is partly related to the widespread and often unpredictable distribution of lymph node metastases. This has lead to interest in the use of sentinel node mapping techniques to improve the accuracy of lymphadenectomy. FI has been shown to be feasible in detecting lymph node drainage from the esophagus in several small series involving peritumoral injection of ICG.[14–17] Although still investigational, proponents of this technique have noted that the potential to improve lymph node dissection either by allowing a more targeted, less morbid approach to node removal or alternatively by ensuring a radical dissection encompasses all relevant nodal stations. Whether either approach will result in improved patient outcomes remains to be seen.[18]

PREVENTION OF THORACIC DUCT INJURIES

Lastly, thoracic duct injury remains an infrequent but persistent risk after esophagectomy.[19] Although the duct has well-known anatomic landmarks, it is frequently not visible in the operative field, especially in obese patients, making avoidance of injury difficult, as well as repairing once injury has occurred. FI has the potential to allow surgeons to prophylactically identify the thoracic duct intraoperatively and to ligate the duct for chyle leaks after esophagectomy, both in the chest[20] and in the abdomen.[21,22] In reported cases ICG was either injected into the small bowel mesentery or into the bilateral inguinal regions, which allowed surgeons to identify and ligate ducts that were otherwise impossible to precisely locate. Whether this targeted approach is more effective than traditional mass ligation based on anatomic landmarks is unknown at the present time.

HOW THE AUTHORS DO IT

The authors routinely use ICG FI to evaluate the perfusion of the gastric conduit and to select the optimal location for anastomosis. Their standard approach is a fully minimally invasive Ivor Lewis esophagectomy (MIE), although the procedure for FI is the same when they use alternate approaches, including minimally invasive McKeown esophagectomy and robotic or open approaches. In MIE the gastric conduit is tubularized in the abdomen but not completely divided from the specimen. At this point if there is any question about the viability of the conduit or the integrity of the right gastroepiploic artery blood supply, ICG may be administered to aid in the assessment. This step is not commonly needed, but administering ICG at this phase does not affect its use later in the operation as it is washed out of tissues within a matter of minutes.

Next, during the thoracic phase of the operation, the esophagus and surrounding tissues are dissected from the level of the hiatus to above the azygos vein and a mediastinal lymphadenectomy is performed. The conduit is then brought into the chest and laid in the proper orientation. The perfusion of the conduit is grossly assessed by observing its color and palpating for tissue turgor. At this point the authors assess every conduit using FI. The standard thoracoscope used for the operation is swapped out for the Novadaq Pinpoint camera (although with the recent technological improvements the entire operation can be done using the newest Pinpoint camera). One vial (25 mg) of ICG is diluted by the anesthesiologist in 10 mL of water and 3 mL of this solution are injected intravenously and flushed in with saline. The Pinpoint monitor allows simultaneous visualization of a standard white light image, the fluorescence image, and a composite image (**Fig. 1**). The speed of fluorescent enhancement is observed qualitatively, and note is made of any demarcated areas of poor perfusion toward the fundus. The process can be repeated after a few minutes if there is any doubt. An end-to-side anastomosis is performed using a circular EEA stapler with an orally placed anvil (OrVil, Medtronic, Minneapolis, MN). Every effort is made to construct a tension-free anastomosis in an area of brisk enhancement, resecting any demarcated and poorly perfused portion of the conduit distal to the anastomosis.

In the uncommon event that there is globally poor perfusion of the conduit or it is not possible to construct a tension-free anastomosis in an area of robust perfusion, several options exist. In otherwise low-risk patients the anastomosis may be completed with a buttress of omental fat and widely drained. The patient is kept NPO for up to several weeks and the nasogastric tube is kept in place longer than normal to minimize the risk of leak. However, in high-risk patients with multiple

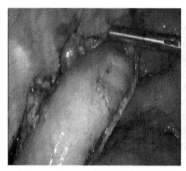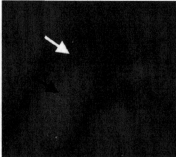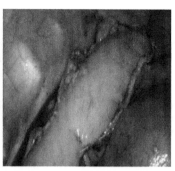

Fig. 1. Different views of conduit perfusion assessment using indocyanine green fluorescence imaging. An area of poor perfusion at the tip of the conduit is identified. White arrow: demarcation between well and poor perfused areas. Black arrow: site for anastomosis.

factors predisposing to a leak or multiple comorbidities such that they would not tolerate a leak, the safest option may be to delay reconstruction until a later time. Lastly, the gastric conduit can be abandoned altogether in favor of an alternate conduit such as the colon or the jejunum. Thankfully the need for any of these approaches is rare.

SUMMARY

The complex nature of esophageal surgery and considerable risk for serious complications encourage surgeons to consider taking advantage of new available tools that offer the potential to mitigate these challenges. Intraoperative FI is a straightforward technique with minimal risk that may reduce anastomotic leaks. The authors have incorporated this technique as part of their standard approach to evaluating the gastric conduit and constructing the esophagogastric anastomosis. Other groups have reported the use of FI to aid in sentinel lymph node mapping and to help prevent and treat thoracic duct injuries. Further research will hopefully help to demonstrate the impact of these approaches on perioperative and oncologic outcomes, but at the current time they remain promising additions to the armamentarium of the esophageal surgeon.

REFERENCES

1. Alander JT, Kaartinen I, Laakso A, et al. A review of indocyanine green fluorescent imaging in surgery. Int J Biomed Imaging 2012;2012:1–26.
2. Zehetner J, DeMeester SR, Alicube ET, et al. Intraoperative assessment of perfusion of the gastric graft and correlation with anastomotic leaks after esophagectomy. Ann Surg 2015;262:74–8.
3. Kassis ES, Kosinski AS, Ross P, et al. Predictors of anastomotic leak after esophagectomy: an analysis of the Society of Thoracic Surgeons General Thoracic Database. Ann Thorac Surg 2013;96:1919–26.
4. Koyanagi K, Ozawa S, Oguma J, et al. Blood flow speed of the gastric conduit assessed by indocyanine green fluorescence. New predictive evaluation of anastomotic leakage after esophagectomy. Medicine (Baltimore) 2016;96:30.
5. Yukaya T, Sacki H, Kasagi Y, et al. Indocyanine green fluorescence angiography for quantitative evaluation of gastric tube perfusion in patients undergoing esophagectomy. J Am Coll Surg 2016;222:e67–9.
6. Campbell C, Reames MK, Robinson M. Conduit vascular evaluation is associated with reduction in anastomotic leak after esophagectomy. J Gastrointest Surg 2015;19:806–12.
7. Rino Y, Yukawa N, Sato T, et al. Visualization of blood supply route to the reconstructed stomach by indocyanine green fluorescence imaging during esophagectomy. BMC Med Imaging 2014;14:18.
8. Shimada Y, Okumura T, Nagata T, et al. Usefulness of blood supply visualization by indocyanine green fluorescence for reconstruction during esophagectomy. Esophagus 2011;8:259–66.
9. Nakashima Y, Saeki H, Yukuya T, et al. Blood flow assessment with indocyanine green fluorescence angiography for pedicled omental flap on cervical esophagogastric anastomosis after esophagectomy. J Am Coll Surg 2016;222:e67–9.
10. Sarkaria IS, Bains MS, Finley DJ, et al. Intraoperative near-infrared fluorescence imaging as an adjunct to robotic-assisted minimally invasive esophagectomy. Innov 2014;9:391–3.
11. Kitagawa H, Namikawa T, Munekage M, et al. Visualization of the stomach's arterial network during esophageal surgery using the HyperEye Medical System. Anticancer Res 2015;25:6201–6.
12. Kamiya K, Unno N, Miyazaki S, et al. Quantitative assessment of the free jejunal graft perfusion. J Surg Res 2015;194:394–9.

13. van Hagen P, Hulshof MC, van Lanschot JJ, et al. Preoperative chemoradiotherapy for esophageal or junctional cancer. N Eng J Med 2012;366:2074–84.

14. Sclottmann F, Barbetta A, Mungo B, et al. Identification of the lymphatic drainage pattern of esophageal cancer with near-infrared fluorescent imaging. J Laparoendosc Adv Surg Tech A 2017;27:268–71.

15. Hachey KJ, Gilmore DM, Armstrong KW, et al. Safety and feasibility of near-infrared image-guided lymphatic mapping of regional lymph nodes in esophageal cancer. J Thorac Cardiovasc Surg 2016;152(2):546–54.

16. Kubota K, Yoshida M, Kuroda J. Application of the HyperEye Medical System for esophageal cancer surgery: a preliminary report. Surg Today 2013;43: 215–20.

17. Yusua Y, Seike J, Yoshida T, et al. Sentinel lymph node biopsy using intraoperative indocyanine green fluorescence imaging navigated with preoperative CT lymphography for superficial esophageal cancer. Ann Surg Oncol 2012;19:486–93.

18. Sarkaria IS, Luketitch JD. Seeing green…augmentation of lymph node assessment with near-infrared imaging in esophageal cancer resections. J Thorac Cardiovasc Surg 2016;152:555–6.

19. Rao DV, Chaca SP, Sahni P, et al. Thoracic duct injury during esophagectomy; 20 years experience at a tertiary care center in a developing country. Dis Esophagus 2004;17:141–5.

20. Kamiya K, Unno N, Konno H. Intraoperative intraoperative indocyanine green fluorescence lymphography, a novel imaging technique to detect a chyle fistula after an esophagectomy: report of a case. Surg Today 2009;39:421–4.

21. Kaburagi T, Takeuichi H, Oyama T, et al. Intraoperative fluorescence lymphography using indocyanine green in a patient with chylothorax after esophagectomy: report of a case. Surg Today 2013;43:206–10.

22. Matsutani T, Hirakata A, Nomura T. Transabdominal approach for chylorrhea after esophagectomy by using fluorescence navigation with indocyanine green. Case Rep Surg 2014;2014:464017.

Best Practices for Training, Educating and Introducing New Techniques and Technology into Practice

Monisha Sudarshan, MD, MPH,
Shanda H. Blackmon, MD, MPH*

KEYWORDS

- Privileging • New practice • New technology • Training • Educating

KEY POINTS

- Key factors to creating a motivated team to deliver new technology include selecting the correct team members, outlining an education plan, identifying resources, and creating a safe learning environment.
- Key factors to implementing new technology in the OR include monitoring of outcomes, establishing a consistent way to deliver the new devices, and post-implementation discussions through quality review, M&M, and formal evaluation.
- In order to offer patients the best and most innovative care, surgeons today must constantly become more comfortable building nimble teams that acquire new technology rapidly and safely. Implementation of such new technology is often multi-disciplinary, and often requires re-training of the surgeon, making advanced surgical training more important now than ever.

INTRODUCTION

The field of surgery has progressed remarkably in the last few decades, including the introduction of minimally invasive procedures, complex endoscopic techniques, and various prostheses (valves, joint replacements, LVADs), to provide a few key achievements **Fig. 1**. The modern surgeon needs to continually refine surgical methods, learn new technology, apply novel techniques, and aim to innovate to provide the best care. However, integrating such new practices safely is a challenging task, especially because a standardized framework to guide practicing surgeons is lacking. This article will focus on providing a guideline for introducing new techniques and technology into foregut surgery practice.

NOMENCLATURE

Knowledge of key terminology including certification, credentialing, and privileging greatly facilitates communication when planning and implementing new techniques.

Certification

The American Board of Thoracic Surgery (ABTS) provides certification through carefully laid out criteria including minimum case numbers and milestones for several standard-of-care surgical knowledge parameters and procedures. Initial certification and recertification are under the purview of the ABTS and generally a requirement by most institutions. However, the ABTS does not provide

Disclosure Statement: The authors have nothing to disclosure.
Division of Thoracic Surgery, Mayo Clinic, 200 1st Street Southwest, Rochester, MN 55902, USA
* Corresponding author.
E-mail address: blackmon.shanda@mayo.edu

Thorac Surg Clin 28 (2018) 573–578
https://doi.org/10.1016/j.thorsurg.2018.07.010

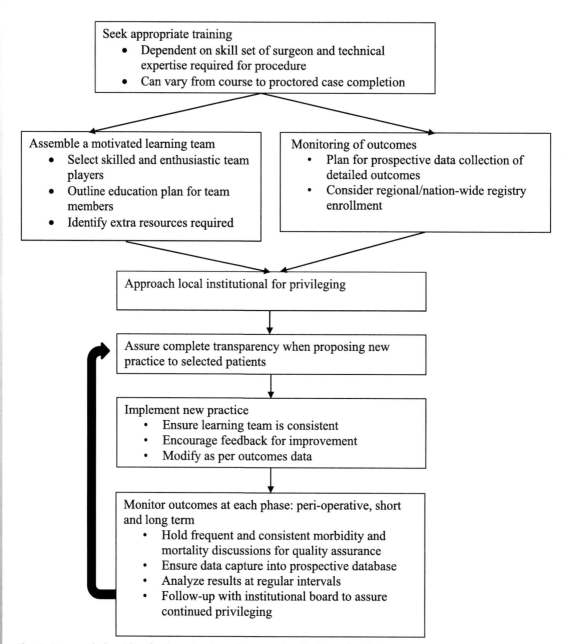

Fig. 1. Proposed algorithm for introduction of new technologies and techniques in practice.

guidelines or credentialing when certified surgeons wish to implement new techniques or technology.

Credentialing

Credentialing occurs at the local institutional level to authenticate the qualifications and practice history of the surgeon. It involves detailed verification of certifications, degrees, training history, and medico-legal issues.

Privileging

Privileging entails the authorization for conduct of patient care services within a certain scope to a physician based on credentials and performance.[1] Privileging occurs at the institutional level, with the joint commission mandating that new privileges should require a focused professional practice evaluation (FPPE) with 4 key elements as outlined in **Box 1**.[2] The evaluation may be timed after a certain amount of cases or a set period of time.

DETERMINING WHICH NEW TECHNIQUES OR TECHNOLOGY TO IMPLEMENT

Success in innovation also requires a careful consideration of the new technique and technology in order to ensure cautious use of limited resources, beneficial results for the patient, and continued patient safety. A few key reflective questions are outlined in **Box 2**. Adoption of new techniques and technology on a societal level is linked to characteristics of the innovation itself, but patient perception, surgeon factors, and industry motivation for promotion have a significant impact on dissemination.[3] Some technologies gain much enthusiasm by the public but in fact may have little benefit. Techniques that are easily adapted by surgeons and teams are more likely to diffuse but may not necessarily influence outcomes or be cost-effective. Finally, industry factors such as marketing strategies, fully funded learning courses, and product discounts can significantly affect diffusion rate. The surgeon innovator needs to objectively reflect on these influences and decide if the new application will indeed improve patient care.

OBTAINING ADEQUATE TRAINING

One of the initial steps after identification of the new technique for implementation is proper training in order to acquire competence and proficiency. New techniques and technology generally lack a quantitative minimum cases and clear milestone tracking as found in ACGME (Accreditation Council for Graduate Medical Education) criteria. Thus, the definition of adequate training if often fluid and depends on the new technology and underlying skill set of the surgeon. In an attempt to standardize such training procedures, the Society of Thoracic Surgeons (STS) experts consensus statement has outlined 5 levels of training[4] (**Box 3**). This nomenclature facilitates communication on the extent of training when conducting and taking courses, in addition to verification by hospitals. However, it does not imply that all new

practices need level 5 or the highest level of training. The guidelines put forth by the Society of American Gastrointestinal and Endoscopic Surgeons (SAGES) on introduction of new technology and techniques also emphasized the depth of training required for the surgeon using a modified device/modified procedure differs greatly from the learning required in implementation of a new device or procedure.[5]

ASSEMBLING A MOTIVATED LEARNING TEAM

The training of the surgeon is an important first step, but training the team to learn and stay motivated for implementation of an innovative technique is also a crucial factor for success. Three key factors have been identified when studying learning teams in cardiac surgery.[6] These include (1) careful team design, (2) motivating the team by appropriately framing the challenge, and (3) creating an environment that encourages communication and feedback. As Edmondson and colleagues elaborate from their study, team design must include members who are not only motivated by the project, but who are good team players, enjoy the challenge of a new situation, and provide frank real time constructive feedback.

Box 2
Choosing a new technique/technology to adopt

How will it impact patient care in comparison to current stand of care (preoperative, perioperative, and long term)?

Will it be palatable to patients?

What is the perceived learning curve for the surgeon and team?

What is the known safety profile?

Does it hold potential to be adopted by other surgeons/institutions?

What are resources required (funding, personnel, equipment, time)?

Box 3
Society of Thoracic Surgeons expert consensus statement on privileging: 5 levels of supervision

1. Certifies the learner attended a lecture or completed a lecture format course. No verification of skills.

2. Certifies the learner completed a course and was assessed with a test or other validation of training and was provided feedback regarding their assessment score. A better model incorporates a minimum pass rate.

3. Certifies the instructor observed the learner performed a skilled and verified completion of tasks. Alternatively, the learner completed a course and participated in a lecture and skills laboratory, allowing assessment of the skills on a synthetic or tissue-based model.

4. Certifies the learner performed the procedure on a patient any clinical setting with supervision with a proctor or preceptor.

5. Certifies the learner performed a series of clinical cases, the outcomes of which should have been reviewed and verified. An example of level 5 learning may be submitting a series of video recorded cases with outcomes to a review committee for verification.

From Blackmon SH, Cooke DT, Whyte R, et al. The Society of Thoracic Surgeons expert consensus statement: a tool kit to assist thoracic surgeons seeking privileging to use new technology and perform advanced procedures in general thoracic surgery. Ann Thorac Surg 2016;101:1232; with permission.

Keeping teams motivated and focused includes framing the situation beyond simply the execution of a novel procedural task. It involves acknowledging that initial attempts will have challenges, but the overall goal is to strive for better patient care and outcomes. Finally, smooth completion of the procedure requires creating an atmosphere that encourages frank input from all levels of the team to problem solve and develop efficiency.

When Edmonson and colleagues studied teams that introduced minimally invasive cardiac surgery, they identified certain favorable characteristics that defined surgeon team leaders. Accessibility to the surgeon was a key feature, with team members appreciative of a surgeon leader available to answer concerns. Surgeons who were open to input from various team members fostered a better team learning environment, and surgeons who acknowledge their own mistakes created an atmosphere where errors can be discussed without fear of retribution.

The authors promoted the exploration of new technology and instruments by arranging a new technology day in the operating room, when staff could ask questions, explore and learn in a comfortable environment.

ETHICAL CONSIDERATIONS

Although a regulatory body such as the US Food and Drug Administration (FDA) is responsible for overseeing the introduction of new drugs, the use of a novel procedure falls under the purview of the local hospital where it is to be practiced. It is the ethical responsibility at the local level, including division chiefs and hospital leadership to evaluate the new procedure and ensure safety and quality via appropriate privileging.[7] One suggestion has been the development of a new technology committee (NTC) that has multidisciplinary stake holders and is separate from the institutional review board (IRB).[4]

Optimal timing in the introduction of new technology is a balancing act between ultraearly implementation, leaving little time to review results, and a delayed response, possibly depriving patients of a useful treatment.[8]

Transparency during the informed consent process ensures patient-centered decision making. A detailed discussion with the patient must address why he or she being considered for the novel procedure, known benefits and risks in comparison to standard of care treatment, and surgeon experience with the new practice. Any financial relationships between the industry and surgeon/institution requires full disclosure.

MONITORING OUTCOMES

Meticulous recording and analysis of outcomes resulting from the new technology or technique allows for evaluation of success and provides targets for improvement. As discussed before, monitoring is part of the FPPE for new privileging put forth by the Joint Commission. At the local institutional level, ideally prospective databases should be set up with collection of carefully thought out short- and long-term endpoint factors. In addition, frequent and regular discussion of cases at conferences such as mortality and morbidity rounds should be encouraged to dissect any adverse issues. If the technique/technology permits, video recording of each case can provide the invaluable opportunity to deconstruct, review, and improve the process.

Institutions may already be part of statewide or nationwide registries that can serve as another resource for monitoring but can also provide comparative feedback on outcomes in relation to other institutions. Proving superior outcomes can be a significant strength to the surgeon innovator during the continued privileging process and to the local institution alike.[4]

CASE STUDIES
Per-oral Endoscopic Myotomy

Per-oral endoscopic myotomy (POEM) is an endoscopic procedure to treat achalasia by performing an endoluminal myotomy. The standard of care comparison is a laparoscopic myotomy with partial fundoplication. At Mayo Clinic, both gastroenterologists and surgeons worked together for privileging, and the POEM program began in 2012. This was recognized as an extension of the surgeons' and gastroenterologists' skill set, and further education was sought in the form of level 4 training that included formal courses, minifellowships, and performing the procedure with a proctor. The clinical practice committee approved privileges after assessing the training, patient safety, and potential benefits. Patients were presented with both options at preoperative evaluation with complete transparency. The first 10 cases were performed as hybrid cases, with the POEM followed by laparoscopic inspection of myotomy. Because these were completed successfully, all POEM cases subsequently have been entirely endoscopic. Favorable outcomes were realized on review of the prospective database. Currently the technique is offered to selected patients, and continual evaluation of outcomes is ongoing.[9] The technique continues to be promoted via proctorship in the operating room provided by coscrubbing.

3-Dimensional Printing

The use of 3-dimensional printing has gained traction in complex surgeries because of its potential to better visualize and plan complicated resections. It has also been utilized to better communicate with patients preoperatively and to plan custom made prosthesis. At Mayo Clinic, the use of 3-dimensional models specifically in thoracic surgery was proposed for the aforementioned reasons in comparison to standard of care, which would be routine review of preoperative imaging only.[10] For the use of this technology, the surgeon did not require any further training; however, the surgeon did work with the 3-dimensional printing laboratory. Privileges were approved by the institution upon review of potential benefits with the use of this technology, with no conceivable safety issues identified. This technology

has since been used in several patients, with a prospective database maintained to document its impact in each case in comparison to conventional planning. Because of the positive impact from this technology, it has since progressed to incorporate degree of tumor response to therapy over time and physiologic activity (or 5-dimensional printing).[11]

Per-oral Endoscopic Plication of the Esophagus

Endoscopic plication has been reported in management of gastroesophageal reflux disease (GERD). Per-oral endoscopic plication of the esophagus (POPE) was proposed to be used for patients with sigmoid esophagus who had been treated for their primary pathology at Mayo Clinic. Standard of care for sigmoid esophagus is variable and can range from observation to esophagectomy. Both gastroenterologists and surgeons worked together for privileging and built on their skills obtained by performing POEM with level 1 training. The proposal was discussed with clinical practice committee members, who provided approval after review of training, preliminary data, and potential risk-benefit for the selected patient population.

Patients with sigmoid esophagus were offered the best conventional treatment or POPE, with full transparency on the novelty of the technique and unclear outcomes.

At the current time, a few cases of POPE have been completed, with no perioperative adverse outcomes. All cases are being monitored prospectively for longer-term outcomes to study the effectiveness of POPE.

SUMMARY

The surgeon innovator is crucial for progress in the field; however, adopting new practices is challenging given lack of standardized processes for implementation. Credentialed surgeons who want to apply new practices need to ensure adequate training depending on the procedure and underlying skills. A competent and motivated team needs to be identified and appropriate privileging sought for the procedure from the local institution. Planning for meticulous monitoring of outcomes via morbidity and mortality conferences, prospective local institutional databases, and regional registries ensures continuous safety and quality surveillance. Patients need complete transparency when being informed about a novel practice, with information on comparison to standard of care treatments.

Increased interest in this subject is emerging, and further funding and rigorous research will provide it with much needed scientific substantiation. The goal is to develop evidence-based pathways that balance innovation, resource management, and patient safety.

REFERENCES

1. The Joint Commission. The who, what, when, and wheres of credentialing and privileging. Available at: https://www.jointcommission.org/assets/1/18/AHC_who_what_credentialing_booklet.pdf. Accessed November 5, 2017.
2. The Joint Commission. Standards FAQ details. Focused professional practice evaluation. Available at: https://www.jointcommission.org/standards_information/jcfaqdetails.aspx?StandardsFAQId=1138&StandardsFAQChapterId=74&ProgramId=5&ChapterId=74&IsFeatured=False&IsNew=False&Keyword=FPPE. Accessed November 5, 2017.
3. Wilson CB. Adoption of new surgical technology. BMJ 2006;332(7533):112–4.
4. Blackmon SH, Cooke DT, Whyte R, et al. The Society of Thoracic Surgeons expert consensus statement: a tool kit to assist thoracic surgeons seeking privileging to use new technology and perform advanced procedures in general thoracic surgery. Ann Thorac Surg 2016;101:1230–7.
5. Stefanidis D, Fanelli RD, Price R, et al. Guidelines for the introduction of new technology and techniques. SAGES; 2014 . Available at: https://www.sages.org/publications/guidelines/guidelines-introduction-new-technology-techniques/. Accessed August 13, 2018.
6. Edmondson A, Bohmer R, Pisano G. Speeding up team learning. HBR 2001.
7. Strong VE, Forde K, MacFadyen BV, et al. Ethical consideration regarding the implementation of new technologies and techniques in surgery. SAGES; 2014. Available at: https://www.sages.org/publications/guidelines/ethical-considerations-regarding-implementation-new-technologies-techniques-surgery/. Accessed August 13, 2018.
8. Sachdeva A, Russell T. Safe introduction of new procedures and emerging technologies in surgery; education, credentialing and privileging. Surg Clin North Am 2007;87:853–66.
9. Renersman JM, Wigle D, Gostout CJ, et al. A novel strategy to initiate a peroral endoscopic myotomy program. Eur J Cardiothorac Surg 2017;52(4):686–91.
10. Dickinson KJ, Matsumoto J, Cassivi SD, et al. Individualizing management of complex esophageal pathology using three-dimension printed models. Ann Thorac Surg 2015;100:692–7.
11. Gillaspie EA, Matsumoto JS, Morris NE, et al. From 3-dimensional printing to 5-dimensional printing: enhancing thoracic surgical planning and resection of complex tumours. Ann Thorac Surg 2016;101:1958–62.

UNITED STATES POSTAL SERVICE®
Statement of Ownership, Management, and Circulation
(All Periodicals Publications Except Requester Publications)

1. Publication Title	2. Publication Number	3. Filing Date
THORACIC SURGERY CLINICS	013 – 126	9/18/2018

4. Issue Frequency	5. Number of Issues Published Annually	6. Annual Subscription Price
FEB, MAY, AUG, NOV	4	$373.00

7. Complete Mailing Address of Known Office of Publication (Not printer) (Street, city, county, state, and ZIP+4®)

ELSEVIER INC.
230 Park Avenue, Suite 800
New York, NY 10169

Contact Person
STEPHEN R. BUSHING

Telephone (Include area code)
215-239-3688

8. Complete Mailing Address of Headquarters or General Business Office of Publisher (Not printer)

ELSEVIER INC.
230 Park Avenue, Suite 800
New York, NY 10169

9. Full Names and Complete Mailing Addresses of Publisher, Editor, and Managing Editor (Do not leave blank)

Publisher (Name and complete mailing address)

TAYLOR E BALL, ELSEVIER INC.
1600 JOHN F KENNEDY BLVD. SUITE 1800
PHILADELPHIA, PA 19103-2899

Editor (Name and complete mailing address)

JOHN VASSALLO, ELSEVIER INC.
1600 JOHN F KENNEDY BLVD. SUITE 1800
PHILADELPHIA, PA 19103-2899

Managing Editor (Name and complete mailing address)

PATRICK MANLEY, ELSEVIER INC.
1600 JOHN F KENNEDY BLVD. SUITE 1800
PHILADELPHIA, PA 19103-2899

10. Owner (Do not leave blank. If the publication is owned by a corporation, give the name and address of the corporation immediately followed by the names and addresses of all stockholders owning or holding 1 percent or more of the total amount of stock. If not owned by a corporation, give the names and addresses of the individual owners. If owned by a partnership or other unincorporated firm, give its name and address as well as those of each individual owner. If the publication is published by a nonprofit organization, give its name and address.)

Full Name	Complete Mailing Address
WHOLLY OWNED SUBSIDIARY OF REED/ELSEVIER, US HOLDINGS	1600 JOHN F KENNEDY BLVD. SUITE 1800 PHILADELPHIA, PA 19103-2899

11. Known Bondholders, Mortgagees, and Other Security Holders Owning or Holding 1 Percent or More of Total Amount of Bonds, Mortgages, or Other Securities. If none, check box. ☐ None

Full Name	Complete Mailing Address
N/A	

12. Tax Status (For completion by nonprofit organizations authorized to mail at nonprofit rates) (Check one)
The purpose, function, and nonprofit status of this organization and the exempt status for federal income tax purposes:
☒ Has Not Changed During Preceding 12 Months
☐ Has Changed During Preceding 12 Months (Publisher must submit explanation of change with this statement)

PS Form 3526, July 2014 [Page 1 of 4 (see instructions page 4)] PSN: 7530-01-000-9931   PRIVACY NOTICE: See our privacy policy on www.usps.com

---

13. Publication Title	14. Issue Date for Circulation Data Below
THORACIC SURGERY CLINICS	MAY 2018

15. Extent and Nature of Circulation			Average No. Copies Each Issue During Preceding 12 Months	No. Copies of Single Issue Published Nearest to Filing Date
a. Total Number of Copies (Net press run)			200	304
b. Paid Circulation (By Mail and Outside the Mail)	(1)	Mailed Outside-County Paid Subscriptions Stated on PS Form 3541 (Include paid distribution above nominal rate, advertiser's proof copies, and exchange copies)	91	128
	(2)	Mailed In-County Paid Subscriptions Stated on PS Form 3541 (Include paid distribution above nominal rate, advertiser's proof copies, and exchange copies)	0	0
	(3)	Paid Distribution Outside the Mails Including Sales Through Dealers and Carriers, Street Vendors, Counter Sales, and Other Paid Distribution Outside USPS®	66	106
	(4)	Paid Distribution by Other Classes of Mail Through the USPS (e.g. First-Class Mail®)	0	0
c. Total Paid Distribution (Sum of 15b (1), (2), (3), and (4))			157	234
d. Free or Nominal Rate Distribution (By Mail and Outside the Mail)	(1)	Free or Nominal Rate Outside-County Copies included on PS Form 3541	34	55
	(2)	Free or Nominal Rate In-County Copies Included on PS Form 3541	0	0
	(3)	Free or Nominal Rate Copies Mailed at Other Classes Through the USPS (e.g. First-Class Mail)	0	0
	(4)	Free or Nominal Rate Distribution Outside the Mail (Carriers or other means)	34	55
e. Total Free or Nominal Rate Distribution (Sum of 15d (1), (2), (3) and (4))			191	289
f. Total Distribution (Sum of 15c and 15e)			9	15
g. Copies not Distributed (See instructions to Publishers #4 (page #3))			200	304
h. Total (Sum of 15f and g)				
i. Percent Paid (15c divided by 15f times 100)			82.2%	80.97%

* If you are claiming electronic copies, go to line 16 on page 3. If you are not claiming electronic copies, skip to line 17 on page 3.

16. Electronic Copy Circulation	Average No. Copies Each Issue During Preceding 12 Months	No. Copies of Single Issue Published Nearest to Filing Date
a. Paid Electronic Copies	0	0
b. Total Paid Print Copies (Line 15c) + Paid Electronic Copies (Line 16a)	157	234
c. Total Print Distribution (Line 15f) + Paid Electronic Copies (Line 16a)	191	289
d. Percent Paid (Both Print & Electronic Copies) (16b divided by 16c × 100)	82.2%	80.97%

☒ I certify that 50% of all my distributed copies (electronic and print) are paid above a nominal price.

17. Publication of Statement of Ownership
☒ If the publication is a general publication, publication of this statement is required. Will be printed
in the NOVEMBER 2018 issue of this publication.   ☐ Publication not required.

18. Signature and Title of Editor, Publisher, Business Manager, or Owner

STEPHEN R. BUSHING - INVENTORY DISTRIBUTION CONTROL MANAGER

Date 9/18/2018

I certify that all information furnished on this form is true and complete. I understand that anyone who furnishes false or misleading information on this form or who omits material or information requested on the form may be subject to criminal sanctions (including fines and imprisonment) and/or civil sanctions (including civil penalties).

PS Form 3526, July 2014 (Page 3 of 4)   PRIVACY NOTICE: See our privacy policy on www.usps.com

Moving?

Make sure your subscription moves with you!

To notify us of your new address, find your **Clinics Account Number** (located on your mailing label above your name), and contact customer service at:

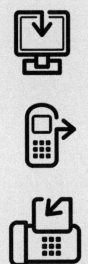

Email: journalscustomerservice-usa@elsevier.com

800-654-2452 (subscribers in the U.S. & Canada)
314-447-8871 (subscribers outside of the U.S. & Canada)

Fax number: 314-447-8029

Elsevier Health Sciences Division
Subscription Customer Service
3251 Riverport Lane
Maryland Heights, MO 63043

*To ensure uninterrupted delivery of your subscription, please notify us at least 4 weeks in advance of move.

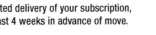

Printed and bound by CPI Group (UK) Ltd, Croydon, CR0 4YY

08/05/2025

01864731-0001